ENERGY
FOR YC

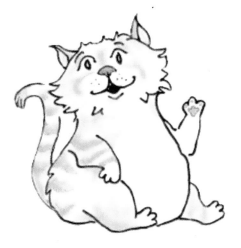

Madison King

An essential guide to working with your cat in a natural, organic, 'heartfelt' way.

Companion book to
Energy Medicine for your Dog.

"A wise and wonderful resource for all animal lovers."

Donna Eden, Author of *Energy Medicine*
and founder of Eden Energy Medicine

All paper used in the printing of this book has been made
from wood grown in managed, sustainable forests.

ISBN: 978-1-78003-875-9

Essential Book Series
Printed and published in the UK

Author Essentials Ltd
4 The Courtyard
South Street
Falmer
BN1 9PQ

A catalogue record of this book is available from
the British Library

Cover design © Author Essentials

I dedicate this little book to
all the animals that have touched my life,
filled it with love, laughter and their own special
brand of animal magic.

I hold each of you in my heart.

Also to all those animals that have not known
love and safety,
may Caroline Cares – Animal Rescue – help find
you a home where you will be cherished and
know loving kindness.

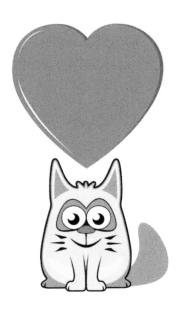

"Madison King's love for and devotion to animals has blossomed into this powerful guide for helping you keep your four-legged friends healthy and happy. Drawing from her vast background in Energy Medicine, Madison not only provides simple, effective tools for keeping an animal vital, she shows you how to attune your intuition to connect energetically to your pet's health needs. It is a wise and wonderful resource for all animal lovers."

Donna Eden – USA
Author of *Energy Medicine* and founder of Eden Energy Medicine
www.innersource.net

"A definite 'must have' for any lover of cats, in fact any animal lover!"

Dondi Dahlin – USA
Author of *The Little Book of Energy Medicine*
www.LearnTheFiveElements.com

"Madison is one of the most fun and inspiring teachers and writers I know and this little book doesn't disappoint – I love it!"

Kim Dowdell – UK
Vision for Living
www.visionforliving.co.uk

"A book to make your cats purr! Madison clearly demonstrates that love is the most powerful tool in animal communication."

Anna Clemence Mews – UK
Author of *What Horses Say*
www.annaclemencemews.co.uk

"Learn how to dramatically change the way you view your cat's health. Empower yourself with natural, effective solutions."

Madeleine Innocent
Dip Hom, MAHA, MARoH – Australia
NATURAL SOLUTIONS FOR VIBRANT HEALTH
http://twolegsandfour.com/

"Now and again a really good book comes along about the joy of working with animals using energy techniques – and this is a great example! Packed full of fascinating and easy-to-use practices, Madison reminds us of the power of working with the loving energy of your heart."

Sally Topham – UK
Author : *Finding the River*
The Energy Self-Help Manual for
Surviving Life's Challenges

"What a great little book, it makes basic energy medicine accessible to anyone – try it, you won't regret it."

Linda Tellington-Jones,
PhD (H)
Founder & President,
Tellington TTouch Training®, Inc
Web: www.TTouch.com

Continued...

"Madison is quite a remarkable lady. She speaks from her heart and only shares what she truly believes in and what works. Therefore her work is trustworthy and practical. Thank you Madison, for putting together such a wonderful book of treasures for our feline friends!"

Mireille Mettes
Developer MIR-Method, self healing method as a gift to the world.
www.mirmethod.com

CONTENTS

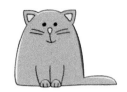

Dedication

Animal stories

Thank you – an introduction

PART ONE – it's all in the preparation

- Are you ready to help your cat? – reprogramme the healer within
- How people sense energy
- 2 secrets to successful healing
- Stress strategies
- Healing from the Heart
- Getting yourself into balance
- Yin, Yang and Heart – the sacred triad
- Heaven Rushing In (thank you, Donna Eden)
- Set your intention
- Coming to your senses
- Your word is your wand

PART 2 – pick 'n mix your techniques

- Pain Relief: stretching, drawing out the pain
- Believe you can do it
- The Hopi Touch
- The TTouch® – Linda Tellington-Jones
- Moggy massage

Continued...

- Tracing meridian pathways
- Timing is everything
- Looking for clues
- How to test a meridian – 3 self-test techniques
- Add or subtract energy?
- Summary of end points on the paws
- Some very strange flows!
- Chakras - general
- Surrogate testing
- Feline Chakra balancing
- Increase your ability to sense energy
- How Nature can sharpen your sensitivity to energy
- Mind's Eye
- Heart spiralling
- The aura – detecting tears
- 'Unwinding' pain through the aura
- A cat in the hand
- Be 'numero uno'
- Polarity issues
- M.I.R. Method – Mireille Mettes
- Touch
- The Divine Codes and how to test them
- Pendulum
- Diet
- Flower Essences and how to test them
- Homeopathy
- Talk from the heart – the cells listen
- Basic energy exercises
- How to Energy Test

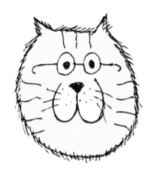

I sometimes hold workshops on ENERGY MEDICINE FOR ANIMAL LOVERS and one of the best parts of sharing the little I know is the feedback and stories. Here are just a couple to give you an idea of what you can expect when you start working with love and energy.

A recurring theme is the improved 'connection/relationship' with the animal, which inevitably brings more joy to both of you. When you work and 'give' to another human or animal, you yourself 'receive' a degree of healing and replenishment – it's a two-way street.

Energy Medicine and my cat

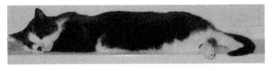

Ingrid and Felix in Holland

My old cat Felix used to always be a bit aloof. He would allow me to stroke and cuddle him, more for my sake than for his own. I love him dearly but a big problem was that he would spray in certain spots in the house. We suspected this was out of stress, but could find no clear relationship with events at home, nor could we find a way to stop him. I was almost ready to give up on it (or go to a cat whisperer) when I bought Madison's book on EM for dogs and started to experiment on Felix.

And found that activating his radiant circuits (a very simple thing to do too!) was the key to his wellbeing. When I tried it the first time he started to purr loudly. He loved it! I kept it up since, with the result that I have a much warmer bond with my cat now. He has become more affectionate, comes to sit on my lap (unheard of before) and his bouts of spraying have clearly diminished.

He just loves Energy Medicine for cats!

Debbie and her farm cat
Cotswolds UK

After attending one of Madison's Energy Medicine for Animal Lovers weekend workshops on the Isle of Wight, I went home armed with some amazing tools. My first port of call when I got home was Streak, one of our cats who had been experiencing chronic itching in his ears, so much so he wouldn't let any of us near him. I employed Madison's technique of figure 8'ing in the aura and he immediately responded to me – I never touched him on this occasion, just worked in the aura over his ears. He stopped moving just beneath my hand, sat completely still, closed his eyes and tipped his head back, nose up toward my hand and began to purr very loudly. The next day he actually came to me and I gently worked on his ears.

This went on for a week and the improvement in the ears is dramatic as is his whole personality, he has become a much more loving cat and now wants to be touched. As well as his ear problem, he had been having digestive problems and would eat ravenously, then immediately bring up his food. He now eats more calmly and is keeping his food down. I feel we opened a 'channel of communication' with him with the energy work and he is not only healthier but happier.

This morning Streak came in after a very frosty night outside and he looked like he wanted me to stroke him. I reached to do so and he crouched away from me, but stood there waiting. So, I started the fig 8's on him again. He then sat down and soaked up the energy. This is his routine now. There just seems to be those days where he doesn't want physical touch but longs for the healing energy and knows he can come to me for it. I am so grateful you have taught this to us in your class. I hope many more people learn of this very simple way to bring their animals closer to them. It is such a gift!

Cow friendly

I employed the Figure 8's on one of our cows, who had a wound that was not healing, was being picked open by the flies. Within 24 hours, it was clean, dried up and healing. Not only did she stand still while I worked in her field, but she allowed me to stroke her head when I finished. This would have been impossible before. Figure of 8-ing animals seems to *calm them and they appear to connect with and trust you more. ...I will never underestimate the power of the Figure 8 now!*

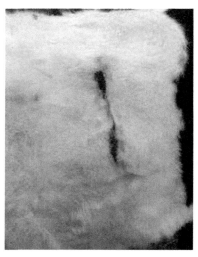 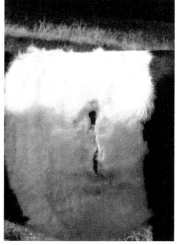

Healing the dizzy lamb

As well as figure of 8's, offering healing energy channelled/flowing from my hands has proven to be a very effective method of treating our farm animals. We had a lamb that was born with a very strange neurological problem. It couldn't stand up for more than a minute or so before its head would twist to the side and it would fall over. This condition persisted and we couldn't treat it with any medications that we knew of. One day I decided to offer this lamb some healing energy channelled through my hands. It was lying down with its head twisted backwards and I just laid my hands on its abdomen and visualised the healing energy flowing to it. I began to feel its gut twisting around as though there were hard knuckles churning around inside. I waited for a few minutes until this churning sensation stopped and then, left the lamb to rest. When I checked on her a few days later, she was skipping around just like all the other lambs with no sign of the previous problem. This was a very good example of how animals are very receptive to healing energy. This was truly a miraculous recovery that even my farm hand couldn't deny.

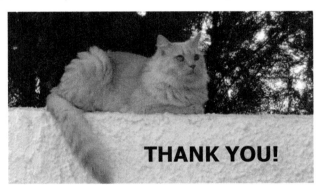

THANK YOU!

Thank you for buying this little book – all the profits from its sales will go to the Caroline Cares animal rescue group founded in honour of Caroline Walsh who sadly lost her battle with cancer in May 2015.

https://www.facebook.com/Caroline-Cares-Animal-Rescue-1653643551557292/?fref=ts

Please tell your friends about it (even buy a copy for some of them) so that we can support Caroline Cares in their efforts to help animals.

I didn't write it alone – an army of pets throughout the decades, farm animals, wild animals, ponies, horses, teachers and friends are behind it; for they are the ones that gave me experience, they are the ones that shared their wisdom and knowledge and I thank each and every one of them. In particular my remarkable friend and teacher Donna Eden who has supported and believed in me for nearly thirty years. Without her I'm not quite sure where I would be today.

I love feedback, so please do send me yours – I can be contacted on: madisonking@hotmail.com
or visit my Facebook page: Madison's Medicine or for an information resource:

or my site:

www.midlifegoddess.ning.com
www.madisonking.com

My grateful thanks to Anna Maria Paciulli for her illustrations and to all the artists at www.Dreamstime.com for some of the other cute illustrations

After the success of **_Energy Medicine for your Dog_** – I had many requests for more 'animal wisdom', especially for cats. So this is the result, it offers you a slightly different approach to working with your pet;

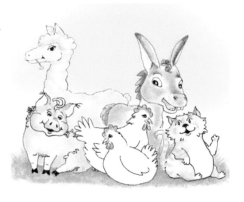

the dog book was very 'hands on', the kitty one a little more 'hands off' with a greater focus on you as the pet owner; a more 'energetically spiritual' approach. After all, as every cat owner knows, cats are totally unique; certainly my little 'princess' prefers to be worshipped (and healed) from afar and a robust spinal flush can only be attempted on rare occasions when requested by her back being presented to me; often lowered delicately onto the computer keyboard, to ensure that I don't miss her request. A regal glance over her shoulder at me, accompanied by a small vocal meow makes it clear that I can drop whatever I'm doing and give all my attention to her back.

Cats respond wonderfully to working in the aura or gently on the body; vigorous stroking can sometimes provoke a 'bite reflex'. However cats are highly individual and I know some who like to be 'roughed up' – just be aware, be sensitive, observe reactions. Be cautious with cats that you don't know.

Read through the techniques and tips and choose to work with those that attract you, which seem to resonate and 'talk' to you in some way. We are all different, we feel energy differently, we sense on a highly individual level and our intuition varies greatly. So it is natural that some ideas will call to you more than others. If they all seem like precious gems in an Aladdin's Cave and you simply can't choose – why not try the 'guidance grid' featured at the end of the book.

Work with a loving heart, be discerning and objectively evaluate results; both immediately and over time. Very often improvements are not noted for a few hours, days or even weeks. Hang on in there... Sooner or later your kitty[1] will show signs of improvement. Often she will surprise you, as animals, unlike humans, do not put up so many 'barriers' and their energies can be remarkably open to love and healing.

You will get a feel for what works well for a particular animal. It will be a combination of the energies of both of you. Most of all, relax, don't judge, have fun and work with an open heart and love... You may be a catalyst for a change that is not obvious at first. Quietly KNOW that you will have helped that animal in some way. Link to a clear healing focus and your pet will tune into, and respond to, the energy of that intention. Science can now prove that animals are influenced by the vibration of our brain wave patterns, of our thoughts, state of mind and mood – so it becomes clear that working on yourself first is essential if you are going to help your animal.

I think it goes without saying, but I will anyway: use common sense and if your animal is seriously injured or you are in any doubt whatsoever – get straight to your vet. Keep searching your area until you find a vet that shares your view of sympathetic integrated

---

[1] I'm talking 'kitty'/cat throughout the book but the reality is that this work can apply to any animal.

animal healthcare. For example, in London an excellent vet who cared for my animals for many years is Richard Bleckman at:
www.roehamptonvets.co.uk

Feel confident that the healing energy techniques I'm sharing with you are totally safe, and can support any veterinary treatment your cat is receiving. The very worst result they can achieve is 'nothing'! Many of these techniques have survived for centuries *because they get good results.* Energy work is easy, natural, organic and absolutely anyone can do it, you do not have to be 'special'. You are simply removing energetic 'roadblocks to recovery', clearing stagnation and congestion; in doing so you allow the 'healer within' to arise within your feline friend. You are returning her body to a 'default' self-healing mode.

K.I.S.S. – I believe this is vital for animal healing – KEEP IT SIMPLE SWEETHEART – the more complicated you make something, the more stress is created in yourself and the animal and therefore the less effective it becomes as a healing tool. Sometimes we feel the need to be complex and take hours to do something that is simple and can be done in a couple of minutes. Let the animals guide you as to how long, what and where. Less is very often a lot more.

Your cat will sense your **loving, healing intention** and the bond between you will deepen: over time, through this work, you will begin to connect with her

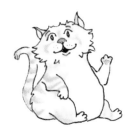

on a much purer soul level. You will find that your intuition overall will increase. Have the courage to follow it and you will instinctively 'know' what your pet[2] needs (and sometimes she needs to be left alone).

If your intuition is a big foggy some days – energy test the 'Guidance Grid' or directly surrogate test your cat. (How to energy test is described towards the end of the book.)

---

[2] For ease of writing and reading I'm also going to use the female gender (sorry boys, no offence).

PART 1

PREPARATION

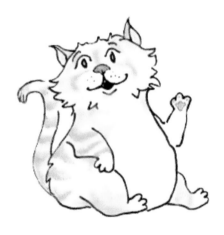

ARE YOU READY TO HELP YOUR CAT?

You can also test yourself to see if you and your heart are open to being a springboard to health for your cat; or is there something, albeit unconscious, that is getting in the way and sabotaging your attempts to help and heal. There can be many emotions at work that make it feel 'unsafe' or 'irresponsible' to help your cat. Sounds illogical? Well it is, but if your 'mini-me' has become mal-programmed around the whole issue of animal 'healing' – then it can create doubt and undermine your efforts.

There is a very simple energy test to see if your conscious and unconscious are united in their desire to help your cat.

Simply say out loud and immediately energy test this statement...

IT IS NOW SAFE FOR ME TO BE OPEN AND WORK PURELY FROM A LOVING HEART TO HEAL MY CAT

Do you test strong? Great, no problem. However, if you test weak it could be that while you CONSCIOUSLY think you want to work from your heart and heal kitty, your SUBCONSCIOUS may not be in agreement! Who knows why that might be – don't try and find a logical explanation as very often one doesn't exist, what does exist is probably an irrational and utterly illogical 'fear' of working with an open heart to heal. It could be caused by a throwaway remark you heard as a child, a TV programme or film or an actual event when you suffered as a result of being 'open-hearted'. That 'wise one within' has become fearful and needs reprogramming, to persuade it that there is nothing to fear, it is SAFE to work in this way with your cat; that there is no danger.

You will achieve this by calming the body (by holding your forehead with one hand and the back of your head with the other) and at the same time repeating (6 times) the statement, smiling as you do it...

IT IS NOW SAFE FOR ME TO HEAL

FROM A LOVING HEART. IT'S FUN, IT'S EASY,

I'M DOING IT AND LOVING IT — all is well

Retest, you should be strong now.

You will need to do this once a day for 21 days to truly reprogramme that particular belief of your 'Mini-me'.[3]

I'd also say, **let go of ego and judgement;** healing does not come because of you but it comes through you, you are merely a conduit or a 'jump start'. Free

---

[3] MINI-ME is a name I give to the 'wise one within' that is beyond your conscious control, it is an area that often operates totally unconsciously. Get Mini-me on board and your efforts will be supported rather than sabotaged.

yourself from expectations, retain a humble trust that what is needed is given and received.

Talking about conduits, I remember when I first started working with energies and the whole concept of being an open conduit... Well, when I tuned in, all I could get was an old green plastic garden hose – no 'celestial streaming' or angelic chants, just a common old hose – and it's remained with me for all these years. I've now become quite fond of it.

So, **humility, integrity and trust go along with loving intention** to form a powerful healing formula and a pathway to health.

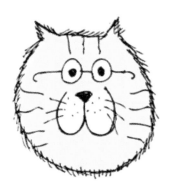

Marcel Proust said: *"The real voyage of discovery consists not in seeking new lands but in seeing with new eyes"*.

A good exercise to begin with is to sit quietly and look at your cat with different eyes, really look at her, how she sits, moves, reacts; look into her eyes, blinking slowly which is considered in feline society as 'friendly', whereas a direct unblinking stare is confrontational. Do you feel a connection? It may surprise you how you will feel an enhanced understanding of what she is and what she needs. You may even find pictures coming into your mind's eye as she communicates with you.

So open your eyes and truly 'see'. The vocabulary we apply to ourselves applies to our cat companions too: e.g. stress, anxiety, strict, loneliness, anger and confusion.

You don't have to diagnose exactly what is wrong – you will be treating the cat holistically, as a 'whole' – after all, everything is connected. This lifts an enormous weight off your shoulders – you are simply helping the animal return to a healthy default mode and in doing so, helping her inner healing ability re-connect to its full potential.

But before we go further, let's take a moment to look at YOU... As a life companion, your cat will be close to you, there will be a true connection and because of this, your cat may be **mirroring** something that YOU need to address. Often it is the owner, not the pet that needs attention. She may be simply trying to catch that attention.

As I said before, healing can more often than not be a **two-way street**. We have all heard of studies that demonstrate that keeping an animal helps reduce blood pressure and stress and even lower cholesterol levels. Sometimes a much more personal healing may be exchanged. A beautiful example of this is when my mother was looking after my three cats for me while I was in the USA. My mother was in considerable pain and one of the cats, Boris, with whom my mother had a particularly close bond, came and sat on the lawn, staring through the French doors at my mother who was mesmerised by the look and the feeling of a loving connection she had never felt before – Boris continued to stare at her and over the next 20 minutes all my mother's pain left her body. My mother was very down-to-earth, but she did admit she felt Boris had deliberately healed her pain.

Sadly sometimes we can't heal our beloved animals, but we can be with them and give them **comfort through the transition**. I have done this with my own animals. In fact with Boris (mentioned above). He lived to the grand old age of 14 (old for a Persian) and one evening I looked at him and just 'knew' he was going to pass – there was no outward sign, but I felt he wanted me to know that he was going to leave; he had come onto this earth plane to help me and support me in learning a lesson and now he was going.

He loved to sneak into the airing cupboard and sit on the towels, so I took two of the big white fluffy towels and laid them out on the bed, he jumped up and laid down and I stroked him and talked to him during the evening. His passing was so peaceful I thought I'd missed it, he was content and ready to pass. I hated the thought of him going but made sure that I 'gave him permission' to leave me. So often our love tethers our animals to this life and makes it hard for them to leave. However difficult it is for you to say the words, an act of love is to say:

Thank you for being my companion for all these years: I forgive you for being naughty, please forgive me for sometimes being selfish or thoughtless.
I release you, I let you go with my love and thoughts forever – go in peace. I love you.

I would mention here that if your cat does pass over, show the body to any companion cats. This stops them looking for her, thinking she is still around somewhere.

Just quietly 'being' with an animal as it passes can bring comfort as I witnessed recently in the American Funduk in Fez[4], a charity set up to offer free equine care to the inhabitants of Fez. A young foal was gravely ill and was lying on the fresh straw in the stable, held in the arms of one of the volunteer helpers – you could see and sense the comfort the foal had with the loving contact and she passed peacefully, literally in the woman's embrace.

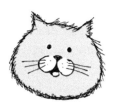 Don't leave it until your cat is ill – working with her in a healing way will **prevent** a lot of dis-ease and enhance greatly your enjoyment of each other. We do need to keep a close eye on our feline friends.

4

http://www.americanfondouk.org/?referrer=https://www.google.com/

They are still 'wild at heart' but we have insisted they live a domesticated life, this can go against their DNA and create problems over time. Often they are bored, lacking stimulation, physical exercise and freedom... and no, contrary to recent reports, I don't believe they are plotting to kill us! They will be however, very sensitive to your mood and the atmosphere in your house and if things are going wrong on that level (grief, anger, fear, pain, loneliness etc.), your animal may suffer. After all, our energies expand out from our bodies and blend with those sharing our space so your emotional disturbance can become your animal's problem too: it can then bounce back on you if you are particularly bonded, so we have an **energetic ping pong** going on. Healing can help return both of you to default.

There are no boundaries to what you can achieve when working with animals, only the limitations you place there yourself.

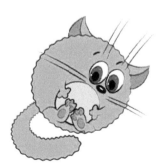

E=mc2

Energy = everything!

Heal the energy = heal everything!

Professor William Tiller at Stanford University said: *"Future medicine will be based on controlling the energy in the body"*.

Energy really is the final frontier in healing, we have come a full circle, our **ancestors were energy healers** and we are now remembering and returning to this ultimate form of healing. What enhances our self-healing also enhances our cat's.

You may be new to energy work and feel a bit sceptical, but I encourage you to relax and open your mind. Think of this: **you can't see the wind, you can't see electricity but both are there**. You witness the presence through the end result: a breeze against your skin, a light bulb turning on. Energy is the same, you may not be able to see it, feel it, touch it, smell it, taste it – but it is there and in time one of your senses will awaken to it and you will 'know' with every cell of your body that energy exists. Learn to trust that 'knowing' however it presents itself to you.

Energy is 'sensed' differently by different people; some see, some feel through their fingers, some have a 'gut feel' and some even taste or smell energy. Let it arrive, let your 'sense' emerge naturally, don't try and force anything – it will come.

With **practice comes confidence** and as your confidence builds you feel more, you are more relaxed and the whole healing process begins to flow and you enter the 'upward spiral' of simply knowing.

ANYone can do this, you do not have to be 'special' in any way, shape or form. We've just forgotten how to do it, but it's in our very DNA to heal each other, we are programmed with this wisdom within.

Working with your cat will simply help you to 'remember'.

THE TWO SECRETS TO SUCCESSFUL HEALING

1. **DEAL WITH STRESS** in yourself and the animal.

2. **WORK FROM THE HEART** with the focussed desire to make a difference... not from ego but from unconditional love and from the soul. The essence of healing is LOVE. It really does throw open the door to recovery – it's as simple as that. The difficult part is getting yourself 'out of the way'.

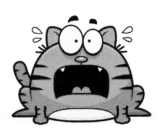

Like many others, Dr Bruce Lipton[5] believes that **95% of all illness and 'dis-ease' is linked to stress** i.e. it is either caused, or exacerbated, by stress. So it goes, that if you can manage stress you can manage illness. We do a lot of work with Triple Warmer in 'human energy medicine', which is the pathway of energy that responds directly to stressful situations. That work applies to animals too.

---

[5] The Biology of Belief – www.brucelipton.com

What is stress to one person is nothing to another and in actual fact it could even be a positive stimulus. It is not so much the 'stressor' it is more **how you (or your cat) responds** to that situation or thought, does it evoke emotions such as frustration, fear, anger, anxiety?

So taking Mumkin my cat to the cattery evokes no stress in her (or me), she loves it and I know she is loved, looked after and most of all, safe. However, to another cat it may be a serious stressor... Their responses to the same situation are different, they have different associations and so will their owners.

Stress is natural.
Fight or Flight is natural.
What is NOT natural is when the fight or flight response is permanently turned on in a human or an animal.
If this happens, stress reactions build up in the body and sooner or later the 'weakest link' will break, things start going wrong, symptoms appear and 'dis-ease' rears its ugly head.

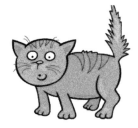

Basically what happens is...

THE STRESSOR appears and Triple Warmer will perceive it to be a true threat to survival. Often this is a psychological threat and not 'real' at all: an irritating boss as opposed to a sabre-toothed tiger. A trip to the cattery not a kitty killing monster! However illogical, however 'in the mind' – it is very real to the body which will react accordingly.

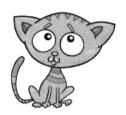

THE HYPOTHALMUS responds, it sends out some 900+ signals (orders) to the body that there's an emergency and to shut down all but the most necessary functions, so that energy is freed up to fight the threat.
(Think of it as: all hands on deck).

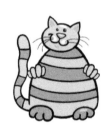

Because all hands are on deck, **THE SYSTEMS** are left vulnerable, which is fine if the stressor is there just for a few minutes e.g. sabre-toothed tiger or kitty killing monster attacking... Not such a good idea to hang around on deck for 5 years.

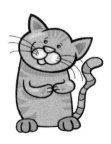

EXTENDED TIME in this mode and the body begins to go out of balance and form destructive energy patterns, so what was designed to save life is now threatening it – even if you do have nine.

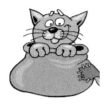

SYSTEM MALFUNCTION occurs as they are deprived of basic maintenance and repair and begin to break down. As all hands are on deck nobody is looking after the basic machinery.

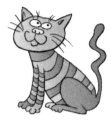

MULTIPLE LAYERS now appear alongside the original stressor and the destructive effect is amplified.

You can see clearly how this cycle feeds on itself, be it in your own body or your cat.

So how do we get on top of stress, how do we 'manage it'?

Firstly, **common sense**: identify the stressor that is causing the problem in the first place – can it be removed? Can the cat's attitude be changed towards it? Can the stress response be switched off safely?

Remember what is stressing an animal may be totally unstressful for you – retain an open mind. Sit and consider, tune in and look through the lens of life from your animal's perspective not your own. What's that wonderful Native American saying? "Try and walk a mile in their paws".

If we can persuade Triple Warmer to release its control, then the Hypothalamus stops issuing the stress response 'orders' – the hands can leave the deck now and this will allow all the other systems in the body to return to normal functioning, maintenance and balance can therefore be more easily achieved, immunity restored and self-healing and repair enhanced.

STOP THE STRESS RESPONSE IN YOUR CAT
STOP THE PROBLEM
START TO HEAL

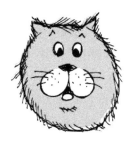

At the end of the day it is the IMMUNE SYSTEM that heals or 'cures'. **Miss Immunity** is the true star of the show but she needs to come out of the shadow of Mr Triple Warmer to be able to do her star turn. We have to reduce stress and loosen Triple Warmer's grip, calm him down so he stops taking energy from, and depleting, the systems in the body, especially the Immune System. It's all about making your cat and her Triple Warmer feel safe and secure; once that happens, self-healing can take place and any 'healing' you do with her will be much more effective and more easily absorbed by the body.

Our task is to reduce stress in the body to set free energy to repair and maintain all systems.

I want now to talk about **HEALING FROM THE HEART**. It's not just a pretty turn of phrase. The love, or heart, energy that resides in each of us is the most powerful healing tool at Man's disposal. The vibrational healing frequency of pure love is the ultimate healer – be it healing a simple cut on your cat or supporting her through major surgery, it is powerful. Our problem, both individually and as a species, is we are becoming more removed from our inner heart healer.

The question is: how do we access it?

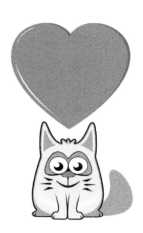

Connecting to your own heart energy will automatically reprogramme you to '**default healer mode**'. In this mode you can be the best complementary therapy for your cat!

Like decorating your home – the finished result is always better if attention has gone into the preparation. It's just too tempting sometimes to skip it. Don't.

HERE'S HOW

- **Grounding and pulling up the Yin**:
  Sit comfortably and close your eyes. Removing the sense of sight heightens your other senses. I want you to now tune into your breathing for a few seconds. Bring all your attention to your feet, connect to them, and feel them. Sense the beginning of a 'frisson' of energy in the soles. Smile as tiny little roots begin to wriggle out of the soles down through the carpet, the foundations, the rocks and earth and burrow down, happily enjoying their new found freedom, into Mother Earth, as they burrow downwards they also spread out around you, creating a huge network of roots. Become aware that any old, stale, tired, stagnant energies are dropping down to your feet, finding their way to the roots and discharging down into the earth, where they belong. Never worry about Mother Earth, she can take that energy and transmute it. When you feel you have discharged all the old energy that is ready to depart, bring your attention to what is surrounding the roots: pure Yin energy, the Goddess, Mother Earth, healing, replenishing, nurturing, calming – feel it connect to the roots, feel it travel up the roots into your feet and up through your feet, ankles, knees, legs, hips and up your torso where it comes to rest in your heart. Sense it and leave it there.

- **Calling Yang down**:
  Bring your hands to prayer position and place them against your chest – in some traditions it is believed that this connects you to your soul. In others that it places you in a state of balance. Bring your hands (still in prayer position) up in front of your face and then up over your head, reaching up to the skies. Keeping the wrists together, open up the hands to form a 'chalice'. Imagine this chalice filling with strong vibrant Yang energy pouring down into it from the skies; a perfect complement to the Yin energy you have drawn up. Bring that Yang-filled chalice down to your heart and feel it merge and mingle with the Yin energy residing there.

You may like to perform Donna Eden's exercise: Heaven Rushing In – again, I'd like to thank Donna for sharing her wisdom and words...

Try and do this out in Nature, perhaps under the stars or a full moon. It reconnects us to the things that are beyond our knowing. This is one of the most comforting exercises in the energy medicine repertoire – you will '*know*' you are not alone. You will '*know*' help is at hand, that you only have to call it in, to ask. It gives you hope when things feel hopeless. I suspect that once you have done it and 'felt' it, you will want to do it daily.

Stand tall. You are preparing yourself to make a sacred connection.

Rub your hands together and shake off any old, tired energies.

Take a moment to ground yourself by spreading your fingers on your thighs, breathing deeply, feeling your feet on the ground and being conscious of your connection to the Earth as the energy pours out of your fingers, down your thighs, and into the ground.

Take a deep breath in, open your arms wide and bring them into a prayer position (palms together) in front of your chest.

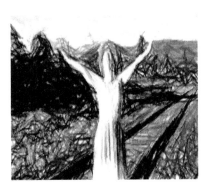

With another deep breath, open your arms wide, lifting them up. Look to the heavens. Reach toward heaven as heaven reaches back to you. Throw your head back, smile and open yourselves up to the heavens.

Release your breath. Bask in the knowledge that you are not alone in this universe and that you are worthy of this blessing from the heavens. You may feel a tingle, a buzz, or heat in your hands. You have been inviting healing energies from the cosmos.

Scoop this energy into your arms and bring your hands into the middle of your chest. There is a vortex here called Heaven Rushing In, and 'heaven' rushes into your heart with healing, with a glimpse of your true nature, and with a peek into who you are in the larger plan. Even when you do not receive guidance or inspiration, know that they will unfold in their perfect time.

Bring your attention to your hands and rub them together again and shake off any old energies then massage open the palms, massage along and off each finger – opening up your hands for the next step.

Okay, so you have now filled your heart with Yin and Yang energy and I want you to consciously stir this in with your pure Heart energy, blending, swirling these three powerful, potent energies together with love into a unique healing mix.

Feel it radiate out over your chest to your shoulders, down your arms and out of your hands and fingertips (that is why we opened them up a little earlier).

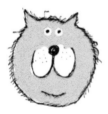 You are now ready to work with your cat, you are a conduit for natural healing energies.

Set your intention: it is the energy of your intention that releases healing potential. One way of focusing intention is 'prayer' or talking to whatever you believe in. You can pray with your cat on your lap or from a distance.

You might consider making a sacred quiet space for prayer in your house or garden – mine is in my garden as I feel closer to Nature there and there are fewer distractions. It is a digital detox zone with no phones or electrical equipment. A candle, some fresh flowers, some incense – make it a place where you can **switch off to the world and switch on the healing potential** inside you. After time, as soon as you sit in the stillness, tranquillity and calm of your 'special space', you will automatically go into a relaxed state of mind and will be able to ground and centre yourself in loving heart energy. It's a great place to distance heal from, to contemplate and don't forget to say THANK YOU a few times too; not only when you have actually received something but also in anticipation. An attitude of gratitude is always a good thing to cultivate.

Being truly in the '**present moment**' is invaluable as a stress minimiser, most of what we stress about is something we did and wish we hadn't or didn't do and wish we had or what MIGHT happen! What minutia is blocking you and your healing abilities?

Here's an old favourite of mine … How to **unclench your mind** with a simple meditation that I call *'coming to your senses'* (as it involves connecting to each of your senses). It is perfect if you are a person who is driven to be 'doing' something all the time and finds it hard to simply sit and smell the roses. It will help you get off the merry-go-round and still the chatter of the daily grind.

This is a gently effective technique that can be done, not only before you work with your cat but also:

A] Before or after your 'Daily Energy Exercises[6] or

B] By itself whenever you feel drawn to it, for the sheer joy of experiencing the tranquillity it brings.

D] When you visit a new place – mountains, sea, building etc., and seek to connect to that place.

E] Adapt it when you are walking, connect to your senses as you take each step: what can you see, smell, hear?

First things first...

When did you last take time to smell the flowers? I have to say that when I am in Andalucía, it is very easy to sit quietly and just 'be' and that is one of the reasons I am here so often. However, I remember when I was in London, I would find myself rushing around, busily getting things done to keep pace with the urban fixation on 'speed'. My diary would be filled six months in advance and joyful spontaneity was a distant memory. My mind could easily become 'clenched' and rigid, filled with useless thoughts, concerns, unfounded anxieties, and numerous action lists and planners. I lost touch with that still/peaceful place inside myself. I became like the White Rabbit in Wonderland! *"Oh dear! Oh dear! I shall be too late!"*. Occasionally, even here in the peaceful Andalucían

---

[6] See my book *Everyday Energy*

countryside, a whisper of that stressful clenching can appear in my life, my rabbit pops out of her burrow and the days get shorter and my action list gets longer and time shrinks and I begin to think of organizing my life in 30 minute segments – I know then it is time to...

COME TO MY SENSES

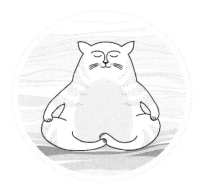

One of the basic principles of working with your energies is for that energy to FLOW freely.

Nothing whatsoever is going to flow through a clenched mind!

How do you 'de-clench'?

Any technique that relaxes and frees the mind will work: meditation, prayer, exercise, yoga – the list is endless. If you are confused and not sure what to do, try this simple technique to exercise your senses. It will gently slow down and stop the merry-go-round, bringing you into the peaceful clarity of the 'here and now'.

It is a great technique for bringing you into the present. Rather than trying deliberately to empty your mind of all the thoughts that plague and pester you, by giving your mind something else to focus on, those thoughts automatically disappear. If they creep back, and they will every few seconds/minutes, don't fight them, just return your attention to the 'sense' you are working. You cannot move forward smoothly in life if you are tethered by the minutiae of small thoughts, each one acting as a guy rope holding you down and preventing you flowing with the natural rhythm of your life and accessing your natural healing ability.

I can hear some of you saying: *'that's all well and good for her, but I don't have TIME to do this or any other technique'* – Don't you?

Then life is ruling you, rather than you living your life.

Look at your schedule carefully, with inspection you will find the time by cutting out something that is not constructive: a little less TV, getting up a little earlier, going to bed a little later, and taking a shorter lunch break, a little less talking on the phone... Think! You can find a few minutes a day for yourself. It will be the best investment of time you will ever make.

When I arrived in Spain, with no landline, no wi-fi or easy computer access, no English television, no shops nearby to tempt me, no nearby friends to see or call, suddenly I found myself with hours of extra 'time'. It became clear to me just how much time we 'fritter' away.

So while being realistic – quietly sit and discover how you can find time.

Okay, so how do you do it?[7] Find a quiet corner in your home or go for a walk in nature and pick a safe, peaceful place to sit.

Ideally sit in the Lotus pose, but if this is not possible for you, find a comfortable position where your spine is straight. A straight spine is vital so that energy can more freely flow up and down the spinal column and therefore out to the entire body.

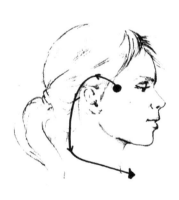

Once you are comfortable, take a few deep breaths, bring your fingertips to your temples and slowly push up over your ears, down behind them until you are on your 'necklace' line (where the neck and torso join). Linger here a moment before pulling your fingertips, with pressure off the upper trapezius muscles. Repeat a couple of times to calm Triple Warmer and introduce a little calmness into the equation.

---

[7] Timings are approximate: you can stay with each sense for a minute or ten minutes – experiment to see what suits you.

1. Now close your eyes and just focus on what you can **HEAR** – keep your breathing natural. Peel back the layers of what is going on around you and you will be astonished at what you start to hear. Remain with this for 2 minutes and if distracting thoughts come into your head don't worry, just gently take yourself back to the sense of 'hearing'. Move past the obvious to the nuances of sound.

2. Keeping your eyes closed, focus on what you can **SMELL** for a few minutes – you might like to prepare for this with a sprig of lavender, mint, rosemary or any smell of your choice.

3. Still with eyes closed, **TOUCH**[8] something. Again, 2 minutes.

4. Focus, for a couple of minutes, on something in front of you and really **SEE** it.

5. If you are outdoors, '**FEEL**' how the environment touches you: feel the breeze in your hair, the sun on your skin, or the rain on your face... Bring ALL your attention to the sensations.

6. Bring your focus to your body, mentally run up it from your toes to the crown of your head and **FEEL** each and every part of it. This is not easy and sometimes when I do it I can't 'feel' a thing, if this happens to you, just remain with it, sooner or

---

[8] You can simply touch your hair, nail, skin, grass, sand or whatever is around you OR be prepared and take along a tumbled crystal, a feather, a leaf – something deliciously tactile, a piece of lavender to smell.

later you will begin to 'feel', begin to reconnect with every cell in your body. If you were doing this exercise with a cat curled up on your lap, you will touch and feel her like never before.

When you have mastered this 'feeling', take it a step further and isolate a particular part of your body and focus your sense of 'feeling' on it. I personally isolate my spine. Leaning forward slightly in the lotus position, to stretch it, not possible if kitty is on your lap. I use my mind to feel along it vertebrae by vertebrae, really experiencing the sensations. If there is stiffness or pain, after a while it will begin to diminish and release. Don't forget your breathing!

End with a classic yoga mudra pose
Sit cross-legged and reach behind your back to clench your left wrist with the right hand, fingers of the left hand straight with index finger and thumb

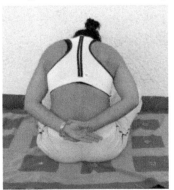

touching to form an 'O'. Close your eyes, lift up and lean forward from the hips so that you feel a stretch but no pain. End with hands over the heart. Tune into your body and focus on letting go of any expectations or barriers you may have to animal healing.

Another benefit of coming to your senses is that by putting them through their paces they improve and ultimately, it may take a long time, once they reach optimum efficiency the other more esoteric senses begin to develop and emerge into the open. When this happens you will find that your ability to **'communicate and connect' with your cat will improve.**

If your cat is nearby – remain in position and figure 8 between you and the animal – maybe heart to heart – it will increase bonding and trust and by osmosis bring a calmness to both of you. You can then proceed with any healing technique you choose to use.

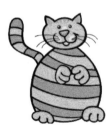

A QUICK FIX

Before you work with an animal, briefly bring all your attention to what you are doing and what you can SEE, HEAR and SMELL. It will bring you right slap bang into the 'present' in a most enjoyable way. You need only do it for one minute. Remember to breathe naturally and smile.

YOUR WORD IS YOUR WAND

Rewinding a couple of pages to 'setting the intention': **prayer is powerful**, so give some careful thought to what you are going to be asking for – you might get it. Focus on love and your cat.

Pray in the positive – it can be written down, spoken aloud, thought quietly or visualised in glorious Technicolor, but make it uplifting; better to make requests such as ***May you return to vibrant health and vitality*** – rather than, *don't get worse, don't suffer or die.* Just saying words gives an energetic power to them so better that you give power to positive words. Two of my favourite authors are:

Dr Emoto[9] (*The Hidden Messages in Water*) his work demonstrated how water molecules are affected, both positively and negatively by words/sounds and as we are c. 80% water (As are our cats) it is a whole lot healthier to talk in the positive. Sadly Dr Emoto died in October 2014 but his work will be continued.

Florence Scovel Shinn[10] (*Your Word is your Wand*). 1871–1940. This title says it all really. Believe me her words are as wise today as they were all those years ago. Her books are being reprinted all the time, they are small (like this one) so quick, easy and inspiring to read.

---

[9] http://www.masaru-emoto.net/english/water-crystal.html

[10] http://www.florence-scovel-shinn.com/

If you are with your pet, speak in a loving way and make sure you are calm and grounded yourself – she needs you to be strong and confident.

Wailing and tearing your hair out is not going to help, in fact it will only serve to confuse and stress your cat. Talk slowly, in a positive, affirming way with meaning and love.

You might like to use phrases like:

- *You are loved*
- *You are safe*
- *You are protected*
- *I love you*
- *I forgive you*
- *I thank you for being part of my life*
- *You will always be a part of me*
- *Whatever happened in the past, it is over (particularly good for rescues)*
- *Whatever changes happen in your body – I love you*
- *I surround you with harmony and peace, with love and joy*
- *Feel my heartfelt love supporting your healing. Trust my love.*
- *I am here and always will be, loving and protecting you.*

Part of your prayer can be **visualising the outcome**, so using the example of a wound: look at it and imagine it closing, healing until it's normal skin and fur. You may imagine 'guides' or 'guardians' helping in this process, wrapping you both in their gossamer cloaks of inter-dimensional magic. Or that particular vision may be a step just a bit too far! It has to be in your comfort zone. End by visualising your cat in vibrant health, totally healed and curled up, purring and content.

End any session with hands over your heart and an attitude of gratitude with the words...

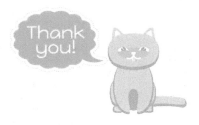

PART 2

TECHNIQUES FOR THE DISCERNING ANIMAL LOVER

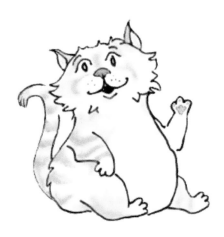

PAIN RELIEF – always where there is pain there will be too much energy congesting the area, so any kind of stretching out and allowing the excess energy to flow and release is going to help. This is one of the basic principles of energy work. If your cat will comfortably allow you to stretch out (gently) an area, it can be beneficial. If she doesn't want you to touch her physically, do it in the aura (the energetic bio field surrounding the cat).

What else can you do if you can't touch the area?

You can draw out the over-energy and pain using this technique:

As with any hands-on technique, rub your hands together and shake off any old tired energy before and after the process and it sometimes helps to wash your hands under cool water to clear them of such energy. I normally wash my hands and hold them under running water for a few seconds AFTER working on an animal or its owner. Massage and open the palms. Do you have a selenite wand? Circle it over the palms of your hand to activate sensitivity in them.

A quick word on Selenite here in case you have not encountered it before. The name selenite comes from the Greek word Selene, meaning moon, so the energy reflects that gentle Yin quality of balance and harmony. In energy medicine it is especially useful to open the palms and to 'comb the aura'; literally comb around your body (or the body of your cat) in the bio field to remove energy blocks and dispel negativity, it restores harmony and leaves a protective energetic 'residue' around the body. It is a beautiful opaque white crystal (gypsum); soft and very sensitive to water so don't wash it or it will disintegrate. A plain wand is not expensive.

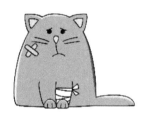

Back to drawing out pain...

Your **left hand** draws 'out' energy, so place it in the bio field above (just a couple of inches) the area that is painful or needs attention in some way.

At the same time place your **right hand** palm facing down to the earth.

The theory is that you draw out the pain through your left hand, carry it through your torso and down and out the right arm and hand where it can flow down into the earth where it will be absorbed.

You may feel drawn to circle anticlockwise, or even figure 8, with your left hand – take notice and do it.

After a few minutes change hands so that the left hand is palm up to the sky and the right hand is over the wound/injury... The left hand is now 'drawing down' healing energy which passes through your body 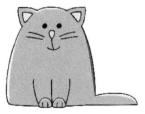 into the right hand where it can balance the area.

If you get the hands 'round the other way' it will still work if your intention is there – working with the principle of left hand pulls out and right hand puts in and balances, just makes it that little bit more efficient.

OK, so you've tried this and didn't feel anything, perhaps kitty even flounced off. So you may perhaps feel the healing way is not for you...

Let go of negative thoughts – **YOU CAN DO IT!** – if you look at the work of Dr Bruce Lipton[11] (*The Biology of Belief*) you will appreciate the power of accessing a loving positive memory or thought**. Negative thoughts keep your body in a state of stress – so change them.**

You may think that you have no negative thoughts and indeed, sometimes they are buried deep, in fact most of the time they are totally unconscious. Hence the importance of reprogramming your Mini-me to loving healer mode and improving your self-belief!

Say the statement and energy test it:

I can activate the self-healing in my pet

If this statement tests weak, then your Mini-me does not believe you can achieve this. To rectify and get it thinking positively. Make a statement such as:

---

[11]https://www.brucelipton.com/

It is now safe for me to activate the self-healing in my pet – I work with an open heart, it is easy, fun and I'm doing it

OR

It is now safe for me to use the power of love and light for healing in the most divine way. I work from my heart and all is well.

There is no need to go into deep psychotherapy for years before trying to heal your pet – just get the energy around the whole issue positive and strong in love, work from the heart and a positive belief you can do it. This creates an energy field that your pet will hook into, before you even begin to do any of the techniques it will be kick-starting the healing process purely by osmosis.

THE HOPI INDIAN HOLD – this technique is thought to have originated in Asia and is known to have been used extensively by the Hopi Indians of New Mexico in their healing rituals. It is based on the belief that you can channel energy and focus it through your fingertips, almost like little lasers over an injured, weak or wounded area, thus directing, more effectively, the healing of that energy. If you could measure the energy (and Kirlian photography can) coming from your hands when you are focussed and giving healing to your cat in this way, you would find that the field increases dramatically!

It's super easy to do.

Prepare yourself: grounding into the Yin Earth energy and pulling down the Yang energy to meet in your heart chakra area. Feel it mix and merge and spill out down your arms to your fingertips and then like 'wolverine' the energy springs out of your fingertips.

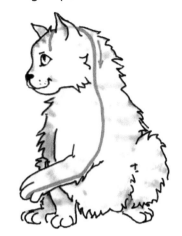

If the animal is stressed, gently going backwards on Triple Warmer (temples, up, over and behind the ears) can calm them down quickly. If they are happy with touch then connect with the body, if not simply work in the 'field'. Hold your fingertips over the skin and imagine all that wonderful healing energy, like little lasers, emerging from the fingers into the cat, wherever she needs healing.

Experiment with where you place your fingers, it is sometimes better to have the fingers an inch or so away from the body, to give the energy space to move. You may feel like touching lightly (like a butterfly).

You can move anywhere on the body, in circles, figure 8's or simply hovering over an area. Whatever draws you.

If there is no specific pain, good general receiving points on the body include: **the spine, the 3rd eye, temples, shoulders and base of spine**.

Touch with love and intention to balance and heal, bring all your attention to what you are doing, **make it mindful**.

Mumkin loves it along her spine. So I simply hold four fingers on one side of her spine, (parallel to the spine so little finger facing head and index finger the tail) four fingers on the other and focus on the energy lasers (the mix of heart, yin and yang) pouring out through my fingertips into her back. When she's had enough she gives me a 'dirty look'; your cat might just walk away.

It's an excellent technique to do over a wound or surgical stitches – it supports cell renewal and wound healing.

T Touch®

I want to introduce you to the simplest T Touch®[12]. I've been a fan for literally decades. You circle one and a quarter times: so imagine starting your circle at 6pm going right round the clock and finishing at 9pm. Adapt the pressure to suit your animal, start off with a gentle touch and increase the pressure. Your 'clock face' will be about an inch in diameter, but follow your instinct. Visit the link below for the full

[12] http://www.ttouch.com/howtodoTTouch.shtml – with grateful thanks to Linda Tellington-Jones for allowing me to share her work.

details; the site is a treasure trove of information. Here is a quote:

When possible, support the body gently with your free hand, placing it opposite the hand making the circle. Maintain a steady rhythm and constant pressure around the circle and a quarter, whether the TTouch® is light or firm, pay particular attention to the roundness of the circles.

After each circular TTouch® you can either move to another spot at random, or you can run parallel lines on the body by making a circle with a little slide and then another circle. Both types of movements induce relaxation and improve self-confidence. By placing your free hand in a supporting position and making a connection between your two hands, this will keep the animal in balance and enhance the effect of the TTouch®.

Most of the time, clockwise circles are the most effective for strengthening and rehabilitating the body, as well as improving self-confidence and performance. However, there are times when counter clockwise circles are appropriate for releasing tension. Practice the both directions and trust your fingers if they are moving in a counter clockwise direction.

MOGGY MASSAGE

Energy Medicine for your Dog includes quite a lot of hands-on massage techniques. Cats may not be quite as receptive to 'massage' per se but I find they tend to like this particular moggy massage called the 'mummy lick'. You are simply imitating what her mum did when she was born and in her first few days.

- With the tips of your fingers stroke from just below the nose, along the side of the mouth then to the ear, pushing gently back (as if your fingers were a tongue) and come off the ear. Some cats love you to give their ears a little massage while you are there!
- You can do one side at a time or both together.
- After a few 'licks', if she likes it continue down to the base of the spine, to the root of her tail and off the tail.
- An alternative ending is to continue down over the shoulders and off the front paws.

My cats have always liked **circling and gently tugging the hair** in random places over the body, Mumkin particularly likes it on her chest. Experiment and carefully observe to see if she likes it and I wouldn't attempt this one on a cat you don't know – you'll get a bite.

We can trace their meridians from a distance, simply by imagining the routes with your mind. Here are the meridian routes for dogs that acts as a guide for cats and other 4 legged friends.

CENTRAL MERIDIAN

(Affects the Yin meridians)

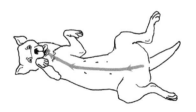

Starts near the anus area and runs straight up the centre of the body to the lower lip.

If your cat has developed the habit of lying in this pose for tummy rubs, take advantage and rub in figure 8's up this channel, always ending with a sweep in the right direction. This strengthens your cat and enhances her connection to the earth and her feeling of 'security' and how she interacts with the world around her. You would pay particular attention to this pathway of energy after neutering.

GOVERNING MERIDIAN

(Affects the Yang meridians)

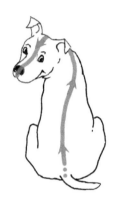

Also starts near the anus (you can start at the root of the tail on the back) and runs straight up the back, over the top of the head and ends on the upper lip.

We naturally brush backwards on this meridian to go with the direction of hair; remember to do one last stroke, in the energy field from tail to head to ensure the meridian is strong.

Lingering over the root of the tail is always a favourite with most cats. I believe it is because it activates this channel of energy along the spine and from the spine itself energy travels out to all organs, so it has a general uplifting effect and gives 'courage' and backbone to a fearful cat. It is also the location of the root chakra which helps her feel safe and secure where she is. Any problems with the spine benefit from this.

STOMACH MERIDIAN

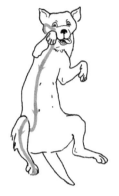

Stomach can be associated with anxiety in your cat. If you do the 'mummy lick' mentioned above and then trace Stomach meridian (albeit in the bio field) it can bring a feeling of calm and belonging to your cat – Useful for rescues, if you have moved house or if she is worried in any way.

* start just below each eye
* drop straight down to the jaw
* along the jaw and up to the front of the ear
* straight down the underside of the neck, chest, abdomen
* flare out at the hips and down the front of the hind legs. Come off the 2nd toe.

ON BOTH SIDES OF THE BODY

SPLEEN MERIDIAN

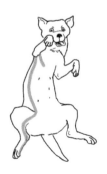

* Starts on the medial toe of the back leg
* Up the inside of the hind leg to abdomen
* Up over the abdomen up to the 'armpit' and down to mid ribs

ON BOTH SIDES OF THE BODY

This really enhances your cat's ability to metabolise and process not just her food but also any stresses in her life. Working daily with Spleen meridian will really boost her immunity. Try this: Go backwards on the meridian once (i.e. from chest to toe) and then forwards in the right direction three times. This eliminates any old stale energy, creating space for new fresh energy to enter the flow. I always think of it as an old-fashioned Chimney Sweep's brush, removing all the old soot from the chimney with that up and down motion of the brush – but then maybe I've been watching too much *Mary Poppins*!

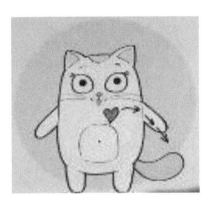

HEART MERIDIAN

* Starts over the heart area

* Runs over the chest

* Down the inside of the front leg

* Ends coming off the lateral end 'toe'

ON BOTH SIDES OF THE BODY

I have talked a lot about working from the heart, so bringing harmony to your cat's heart energy will be a powerful component to enhancing the heartfelt loving bond between the two of you. Try stroking this meridian while telling her you love her and end by tracing a little heart over her heart (3 times).

SMALL INTESTINE

* Outside of the lateral 4th toe
* Up along back of leg
* Over the shoulder blade
* To the bottom of the neck
* Along neck to jawbone
* Up cross the cheek
* Past the eye
* Ends just in front of the ear

ON BOTH SIDES OF THE BODY – as you can imagine, this is a favourite to work if your cat has any aches and pains in the shoulder area as well as a digestive upset.

BLADDER MERIDIAN

* Begins between the eyes
* Comes up over the skull
* Down back of neck to shoulder blade
* Spread palm out so it covers a dual pathway down the side of the spine
* Becomes one again at the pelvis
* Runs down the back of the hind leg
* At the 'heel' comes round to the outside
* Comes off the outside of the 4th toe (back leg)

ON BOTH SIDES OF THE BODY

Definitely one to work if your cat is a rescue and feeling pretty hopeless about life. With Governing meridian, this is a must for any spinal problems.

KIDNEY MERIDIAN
Begins under the paw
Runs up inside leg
Up the abdomen
Up the chest
Ends at base of the neck

ON BOTH SIDES OF THE BODY – Excellent meridian when your cat is in a state of FEAR, so again, excellent for rescues. Firework night: work kidney, stomach and triple warmer to help calm her.

PERICARDIUM
* Starts at the chest area near the heart
* Runs down to the elbow
* Down inside of foreleg
* Come off the 2nd toe

ON BOTH SIDES OF BODY

The pericardium protects the heart so you would work with this meridian when the cat is going through any 'sadness' –

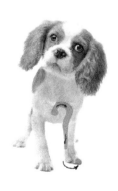

missing an owner, feeling alienated in any way, loss of sibling etc. The meridian also partners Triple Warmer so can be associated with stress – one of my cats absolutely adored being stroked along this meridian – see how yours reacts.

TRIPLE WARMER

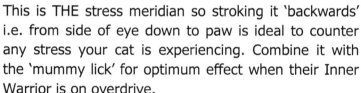

* Begins at outside of the 4th toe (front leg)
* Runs up the leg to elbow
* Over the shoulder
* Up the side of the neck
* Behind the ear
* Over top of ear
* Ends at temples/side of eye

BOTH SIDES OF THE BODY

This is THE stress meridian so stroking it 'backwards' i.e. from side of eye down to paw is ideal to counter any stress your cat is experiencing. Combine it with the 'mummy lick' for optimum effect when their Inner Warrior is on overdrive.

GALLBLADDER

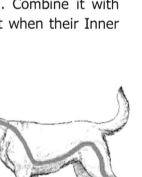

* Starts at the outside corner of the eye
* Move back to the ear
* Move forward to the temples
* Move back over the ear

- Move forward over the forehead
- Back on the forehead
- Down the neck
- Down to the shoulder
- Over the side of the body to the pelvic area
- Down the outside of the back leg
- Comes off 2nd toe

BOTH SIDES OF THE BODY – if the beginning of the meridian seems all a bit too confusing, try this... with your cat sitting in front of you, start with a mummy lick on both sides and then with open palm stroke up the temples, up over the ears down behind the ears, over the shoulder, down the rib cage and off the back paw... What could be simpler? I find they quite like this one with a firmer pressure than used on the other meridians. It is excellent if you have a grumpy cat that is angry with the whole world!

LIVER MERIDIAN

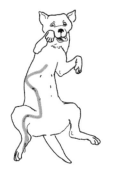

- Begins at the dew claw on back leg
- Runs up the inside of the leg to pelvic area
- Fares out to the side
- Comes back in and meets at lower chest area

BOTH SIDES OF THE BODY. I don't think cats ever get angry at themselves but if they do feel a bit 'liverish', this works a treat. The liver has so many different functions so balancing is essential to optimum health and body flexibility.

LUNG

* Starts over the lung area
* Runs down inside of front leg
* Ends coming off the dew claw

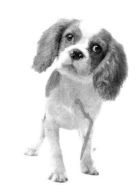

BOTH SIDES OF THE BODY – lung is often associated with grief and sadness. If you live in the city with all its pollution, your cat may benefit from working this meridian. Breathing problems benefit.

LARGE INTESTINE

* Tip of the 1st toe (medial) of front leg
* Up the inside of the leg
* Move out to the elbows
* Up over front of shoulder
* Up side of neck
* Along top lip
* Ends at side of nostril

BOTH SIDES OF THE BODY – to help digestion and elimination.

TIMING IS EVERYTHING!

Every pathway is associated with a 2 hour time 'slot', which can provide a clue – does a particular time slot correspond to a physical symptom or behavioural quirk of your dog? If it does then maybe by balancing the associated meridian by tracing or flushing the pathway (stroke backwards on the pathway once and then forwards three times) you can influence the physical or emotional aspects. So, for example if your cat displays strange behaviour at midnight, you might try stroking the Gallbladder meridian (11pm–1am time slot) and see if it helps.

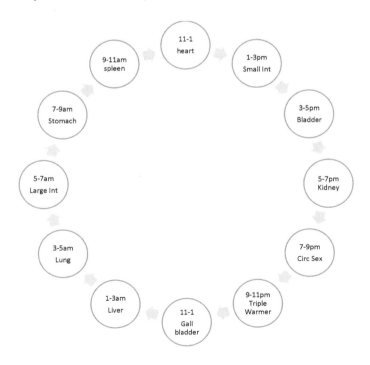

Also, where does the physical problem occur? What meridian is it on? Does it clearly sit on a pathway of energy? Try working with that meridian (by 'working with', I mean resetting the meridian: **tracing backwards x 1 forwards x 3)** and see if it helps. Pain is nearly always associated with OVER energy, too much energy on a meridian; so tracing it backwards removes some of that OVER energy and can reduce pain.

Energy needs to flow around this 'wheel' with no blockages; when they do occur the energy becomes stagnant and tired and can cause problems and pain. Think of them as roadblocks on the motorway to recovery. Simply stroking all the meridians in sequence can help remove the blocks.

By regularly (two or three times a week) tracing your cat's meridians you can help prevent imbalances moving into the physical from the energetic and if there is already a physical problem, by getting the energy moving you are allowing space for the cat's inner healer to function to her optimum level.

LOOKING FOR CLUES

Let's take an example, after looking for the obvious, go a bit deeper:

Say Mumkin has a stiff back leg and hip area, for no obvious reason. First of all, what is stiffness associated with? Wood element. So I would immediately suspect Wood (liver and gallbladder).

You might choose to surrogate test the meridians to see if they are in balance or not. (see below)

I can then look at what meridian runs through or close to the painful area and in this case it would be Gallbladder on the outside and Liver on the inside leg (in another example it might be another element) – so I would definitely be balancing Gallbladder and Liver by tracing either on her body or in the bio field over it.

I might look for further clues, has she been more grumpy lately? Remember GB is associated with outwardly directed 'anger'. Does it get worse at a particular time of day? In the case of Wood, I would be looking at 11pm–3am.

I might also suspect Bladder, Stomach, Kidney and Spleen which all run through the back legs.

HOW TO TEST A MERIDIAN

I might surrogate test the suspect meridians by holding the end point of each – focussing with my mind on the route it takes and testing. Don't worry if you are not quite sure of the spot, intention is king in energy medicine. Energy follows intention (and your hand).

If you don't have a surrogate you can self-test the meridians:

Simply hold the end point (either beginning or end, it doesn't really matter which one, go for the one more easily located). Set the intention that you are testing the cat's meridian and perform a 'self-test' of your choice.

I suggest you try each of the self-tests below and see which one you find the most effective, comfortable and the easiest, then stick with that one and practise, practise, practise.

It has to be said you can influence these tests if you choose to. Be sure that you are feeling as objective and neutral as possible. Tell yourself you are seeking the truth, any interference would only be a form of sabotage and not help your cat.

THE PENDULUM TEST

You will be using your body as a pendulum: stand, barefoot if possible, feet solidly on the floor, not too far apart, knees unlocked, take a deep breath, set the intention that you want an honest dialogue with yourself.

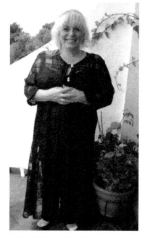

Place one hand over your solar plexus and the other hand over the first.

Tuck your elbows into your sides.

Close your eyes and say "*my name is Minnie Mouse*". Now, does your body sway forward or backward?

Repeat the test but this time saying *"my name is (your name)"* – what happens?

Normally the body will sway forward toward the truth or a substance that is strong/positive and easily metabolised and backward i.e. away from one that is weak/negative, does not suit the body chemistry, or an untruth. If a meridian, organ etc., is in balance it will sway in the strong/positive direction.

It will either be attracted or repelled. You will sway forward or backward.

However, rules are always made to be broken and some people buck this trend. You may even vary occasionally. By using the Minnie Mouse test you can establish your personal weak and strong sway for that day.

Testing your cat's meridian requires you to hold one end point, your other hand will remain over your solar plexus. You will test first on one side of the body and then the same meridian on the other paw.

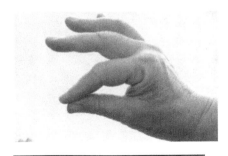

THE STICK TEST

The stick test was shown to me by Dr Michael Burt ND[13]. It is so discreet it can be used anywhere, anytime. In fact, a

---

[13] A truly remarkable naturopath in London – www.brabandhouseclinic.co.uk

friend of mine who has been using it for years, can test the menu at any restaurant she visits, using this technique. Nobody realises she is selecting the healthy choice for her body.

Centre yourself and take a deep breath, relax and rub the pads your index finger and thumb together, naturally, no real pressure. Now, as before, say "my name is Minnie Mouse" and observe what happens, do the fingers slide together more easily, or do they feel a little more 'sticky'? Repeat using your own name and observe what happens.

If you feel a marked difference, then this is a great test for you to practise as it is so easy and unobtrusive. Normally sliding more easily indicates a positive and feeling more friction, a certain 'stickiness' indicates a negative.

THE QUAD TEST

Testing the quadriceps muscle is not quite as convenient, but it is easy and reliable: sit straight on a chair, with feet firmly planted on the ground in front, the chair should neither be too high nor too low. Lift one leg slightly off the chair. Now, with the heel of your hand, press down on that knee, while the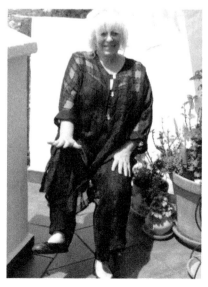

knee resists. If the leg stays locked take it as a strong result but if the leg goes down easily then it is a weak result.

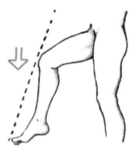

For any test you need to be grounded and objective – I often say to myself: ***"I seek the truth and what I do with that truth is my choice, but it would be interesting to know xyz"*** — it helps me keep centred and therefore aids accuracy in testing.

As with the surrogate testing you can check you have a clear yes/no by testing a true statement such as "*My name is and say your name*", it should test strong, whereas an obviously untrue statement such as "my name is Minnie Mouse" would test weak.

ADD OR SUBTRACT?

If a meridian tests 'weak'; **reset by tracing forwards and retest** – it should now test strong. If it is still weak that could indicate that the pathway has TOO much energy on it, often the case when pain is involved. It definitely didn't want the extra energy you were bringing in by tracing. It will however benefit from tracing BACKWARDS on it. So, do that and test – it should now be strong as you have taken some of that over energy out and restored it to a balanced flow and you have one happy meridian.

To summarise: if a meridian tests strong when you trace it, it didn't have enough energy in it so responded well to you adding some. If it tests weak when you trace it, it probably has too much energy and definitely doesn't need any more added. It would respond well and test strong if you took some of that excess energy out of it by tracing backwards.

TO SUMMARISE THE END POINTS ON THE PADS:

Front legs

* THE EQUIVALENT OF OUR THUMB (**dew claw**) – Lung
* Forefinger (medial) – Large Intestine
* Middle finger – Pericardium
* Ring finger – Triple Warmer
* Little finger – Heart and Small Intestine

Back legs

* Central pad – Kidney
* Medial 1st Spleen and Liver
* 2nd – Stomach
* 3rd – Gallbladder
* 4th – Bladder

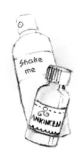

Rubbing a little diluted flower essence on the paws can help heal emotions. They do not smell. You can also rub a few drops on your hands before tracing the meridians. Cats are very sensitive to smells so essential oils or anything smelly can be a turn-off to them.

SOME VERY STRANGE FLOWS!

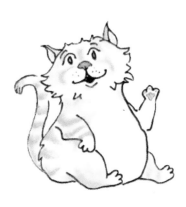

I love the ancient 'strange flows' of energy and they translate beautifully on our cats. They are also called the Extraordinary Vessels in Traditional Chinese Medicine. Donna Eden calls them Radiant Circuits as the energy they carry is indeed pure radiance. The reason I love using them with my cats is that they are a very spiritual energy and therefore resonate well with the slightly 'mystical' aspect of our cats, a quality deeply appreciated by some ancient cultures such as the Egyptians.

Little is known here in the West but these are used extensively in TCM (Traditional Chinese Medicine) in the East. They appear to predate meridians and are the first energy circuit to appear in the developing foetus – they are truly ancient flows of energy that perhaps, in our distant ancestors, flowed freely through the body; some, over time however, repeatedly began to serve specific organs – was it these that then developed into what we know as the fixed energy channels called meridians? *Are meridians just Strangeflows stuck in a rut?*

Animals can be far more connected to their 'strange flows' than us humans and respond quickly to working with them; they appreciate that these flows are flows connected to 'joy' and feel good so they naturally gravitate towards that positive energy. Cats, in most cases, deal with stress in a more efficient way than humans do and therefore, in general, are not Triple Warmer dominated, this in turn encourages the free flow of the 'strange flows'.

They help your cat deal with change, they protect using the principle of harmony (they are diplomats not 'special forces') and will troubleshoot anywhere in the body where help is needed. So you can begin to see how very useful these flows can be in maintaining your pet's well-being.

All animals will benefit from free flowing Strangeflows. As you will, and that's the beauty of working this technique, as you balance her flows, yours react too and begin to find their own harmony. You don't even have to know what is wrong with her, the Strangeflows will find the disharmony and work on it.

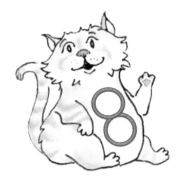

One very simple way of activating the flows is to lightly scratch your pet's back all over, from top to bottom and trace in the 'aura' lots of figure 8's both on the back, tummy in fact **anywhere on the body.** Any size. This will instantly activate all the flows.

Remember when you were a child you drew letters on you friends' backs and they had to guess what you had written? Children all over the world do this. Why? Because instinctively they know it makes them feel more joyful. It will do the same for your cat.

You can also 'trace' the flows. Rub your hands together and shake off any stale and tired energy and place them over the beginning of the flow and slowly move your hands along it. Keeping to the direction indicated until you reach the end. Do it on both sides of the body.

Your hands are like little electromagnetic pads and when you align them, with a loving intent, to a flow on your pet, as you move the hand, the energy on the flow will follow. So you will literally be moving your pet's energy with your hands.

Follow the diagrams overleaf for my 2 favourite flows that work particularly well with cats.

Belt (or girdle) flow. Pull round the 'waist' a couple of times before tracing down and off the opposite leg and paw. Repeat on the other side.

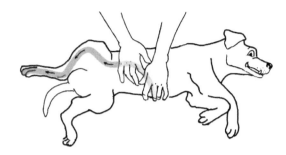

This flow is vital for your cat's ability to balance her natural instincts and the practicalities of being your pet! Good for hip and leg health and a must for digestion and reproductive systems.

Next let's look at one of the most valuable 'tracings' you can do on your cat (and on yourself for that matter). It's called Regulator. That's exactly what it does, it helps her regulate and adjust to any change in her life or any change you are trying to achieve with your work on her.

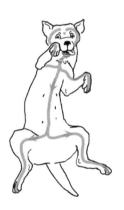

* Start with your hands on her third eye
* Trace round her face to the tip of her jaw
* Down over her windpipe to her throat

- Branch out to the shoulders
- Down both legs hands around the limbs and off the front paws
- Hands off and place on her chest
- Down the front of the belly
- Off both her back paws and give them a little squeeze

THE BACK (YANG) FLOW is loved by all animals: start with a mummy lick, mouth to ear. Teddy Boy Sweep. Circle shoulders. Down the spine and off both legs and squeeze the paws.

CHAKRAS

Chakras can be worked from a distance. They vary slightly on animals but it is the intention that carries the power so don't worry too much if the position is 100% correct or not.

If you are working on the body, you can calibrate the strength of the chakra with a pendulum. Simply hold it above the chakra and see how fast and strong a spin it has.

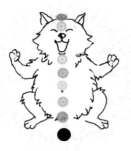

- **Crown** on the top of the head between the ears
- **Brow** over the brow
- **Throat** over the throat
- **Heart** over the heart
- **Solar plexus** on the 'withers'

- ***Sacral*** *chakra over the womb area*
- ***Root*** *chakra is located at the base of the tail on the top*
- ***Earthstar*** *about 18" below the paws*

Chakras 1–6 can be accessed on the spine too and in the case of a nervous or vulnerable cat, it might be an easier way of connecting.

It is said that there is an extra key **chakra on the shoulder** of animals, Margrit Coates talks about it in her book *Healing for Horses*. To me it is as if the heart energy comes out, not only on the spine and under the cat but also to the side to the shoulders. Like the throat, it is linked to and affects all the other chakras. I know my cats love simply being held on both shoulders with a subtly gentle circling of the skin over the muscle/bone.

There is also the **Earth Star** situated about eighteen inches beneath the back paws. This can be useful in re-homing:

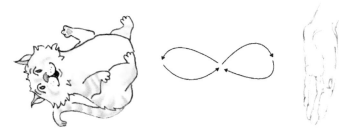

simply bring the palm of your hand to the back paws – draw it back about 18 inches (about 45 centimetres) – close your eyes and try and feel the energy in that area then figure 8 between the back paws and the Earth Star – slowly either with your hand or with your mind's eye – six or seven times.

Focus on the throat chakra because I believe, like humans, animals have the 7 chambers located there so if you work the throat, you are working everything. Simply hold the palm of your hand in the front of the throat and one on the neck – your hands are palm to palm with the throat chakra in between and thus receiving energy from both palms. Work in the aura and if you feel the urge to circle or figure 8 do so, focus is on feeling the connection with the throat chakra.

Now on to **surrogate testing**, an invaluable tool to test any animal.

You can test the:

- **Foods** – is your cat's body processing the food you are feeding her, or is it putting her body under stress? The latter can often result in behavioural or skin problems. Test to determine exactly what foods suit your cat's unique chemistry.
- **Supplements** – optimum dose and frequency.
- **State of the organs** – is there an energetic imbalance in the organs that could manifest in a physical problem (it may already have done so)? If you work the corresponding meridian and retest, the result will tell you if your correction has been helpful or not.

- **Spine and joints**. This is particularly useful for any injuries or stiffness that can often be caused by energy running backwards and ultimately getting stuck in the joints with age. Get the energy moving and you will diminish the pain.
- **Chakras, aura and meridians** – balance in these is essential to vibrant health.

You will need a third person, a surrogate, who effectively acts as an 'energy receiving station'; they will be the link between you and your cat. This may sound unbelievable, but it works.

All the testing is carried out in the normal way on the surrogate, *(basic guidelines to testing at the back of the book, but just think of the surrogate as a cat's extra-long paw)*. The surrogate and cat maintain contact throughout. This contact is most normally a hand on shoulder or head/neck.

Needless to say it is imperative that the surrogate is in balance so that they can act as an effective connection. A simple balance of 3 Thumps and X Crawl is often all that is necessary *(see at the end of the book)*.

Check the surrogate is testing correctly by getting them to make a false statement (such as 'my name is Minnie Mouse') and energy test it – it should be weak. Energy test a true statement (such as 'my name is' whatever the name is of the surrogate) and it should be strong.

You now know the energy is talking to you and in the right way.

So the basic surrogate routine would be...

* *Balance yourself with basic 3 thumps (see end of book)*

* *Surrogate does the same*

* *Energy test the surrogate to ensure they are in balance and you can get a clear test i.e. a clear yes/no response*

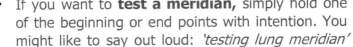

* *Surrogate places hand on the cat. They can be standing or sitting, it doesn't matter*

* *Both of you to be grounded and bring the intention of testing the cat*

* *You introduce the substance being tested anywhere against the cat and test the surrogate (if this is difficult, you can hold the substance against the surrogate with clear intention). Or you may want to touch and focus on a wound, organ, joint or injury*

* If you want to **test a meridian,** simply hold one of the beginning or end points with intention. You might like to say out loud: *'testing lung meridian'*

(or whatever meridian you have chosen) as you test the surrogate

❧ If you want to **test a chakra**, tap over the chakra and test

FELINE CHAKRA BALANCING

As with humans, feline chakra work can be exactly right for problems that result from emotional and hormonal disturbance, so ideal for helping cats through trauma of any kind.

It can be an opportunity to work on a more spiritual level, especially over the heart (and shoulders) chakra area... it's where we connect with our animals.

The actual technique is so simple yet it can have profound results, so don't be deceived by that simplicity.

Place the palm of your hand (normally we start with the left hand as it 'draws out' energy and you want to draw out and connect with the chakra's energy). Slowly move your hand away, gaining a sense of where the energy is, often about a couple of inches – if you can't 'feel' anything, work about an inch or two off the body.

You now start to 'stir the soup' by moving the left hand slowly in an anti-clockwise direction for a minute or two, end by spiralling outwards and then shaking off the hand.

Do the same with the right hand, but this time in a clockwise direction.

End by tracing a 'figure 8' over the chakra area.

Retest to ensure that the balance has indeed bought a balance to the chakra. (i.e. tap the chakra on the cat and either surrogate or self-test).

INCREASE SENSITIVITY TO FEEL ENERGY

Try this simple Qigong exercise that may help you increase your sensitivity and ability to 'feel' your cat's energy.

Sit comfortably with feet resting flat on the floor and back straight. You are connecting to Earth and with a straight back, energy is not hindered, it can free flow.

Place your hands on your knees, palms up.

Just stay there for a minute, breathing gently – calm down.

Rub your hands together and shake off any old, tired energy into the earth. Press the centre of each palm and massage it with your thumb to open it and activate the hand chakras. You can also press with Selenite or crystal wand and if you have a cut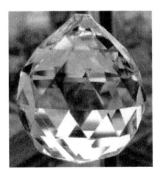

glass prism,[14] spin it over the centre of the palm.

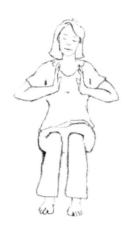

Bring your hands to chest level with palms facing each other about 12 inches apart – arms are bent at the elbow – imagine you are holding a plastic beach ball or balloon in front of you; feel how it supports and pushes and moves under your touch. Nothing is rigid, it's totally fluid.

Stay with this for a minute or two, smile, enjoy it; the less tension the more sensitivity.

Breathe naturally and with each exhalation imagine the energy flowing into the centre of the palm. What do you experience? Observe any sensation between your hands: warmth, coolness, tingling, heaviness, a feeling that the hands want to move out – don't stress it, don't judge it, don't try and make sense of it – just be aware of the feeling.

Start playing with the experience by bringing the two palms closer together and then apart again. Feel that 'beach ball/balloon' expand, contract and come alive.

---

[14] Available in the Energy medicine Toolkit (http://www.theinnersourcestore.com/the-energy-medicine-kit/) or make your own if you have a small cut glass prism ball, simply thread some dental floss through it, knot the floss so that you can spin it easily between your finger and thumb – see my site www.midlifegoddess.ning.com for instructional video clip.

Now move the palm of one hand, it doesn't matter which, over the forearm – what do you sense, how close do you feel like being? Repeat on the other arm. Take your time.

Do this every day for two weeks to increase the sensitivity of your hands.

HOW NATURE CAN HELP SHARPEN YOUR SENSITIVITY TO ENERGY

Lie down on the lawn, feel yourself sink into it, feel the entire weight of your body connect with the earth beneath you, feel it supporting you, holding you, protecting you. Open up to it, do you feel it connecting with you, after all the connection goes both ways.

Trees have life energy fields around them – close your eyes and hold your hands about 6" away from a tree and see what you can sense. Lean your back against the trunk and sense through your spine the energy.

Nature is pure and can be easy to 'sense'. Place your hands around any flower or plant or dig your fingers into the earth; close your eyes to heighten your other senses and tune in.

Introducing Nature into your Sensitivity practice can be a peaceful, enjoyable way to develop your senses. Wherever we live we can find a little corner of Nature – albeit a small roof garden in Central London or the wide open canyons in America or the green lush valleys of Wales or the rugged mountainsides of Scotland.

In the Buddhist tradition, there is a walking meditation technique that can be very useful in connecting with the earth and getting grounded. Stand all, step your left foot forward, then right – but with awareness and slowly. One of the best demonstrations of this is on the following link for Yuttadhammo Bhikkhu:

http://www.youtube.com/watch?v=_IFvablc6EI&list= TL7Kze4qiww04

MIND'S EYE – pineal gland/3rd eye

When you are working with your energies, close your eyes, you immediately boost your ability to access your senses.

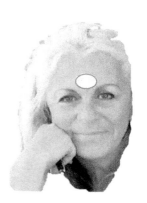

It is said that if you close your eyes, your 'mind's eye' / 3rd Eye becomes more active, you will see and sense more easily.

The 3rd eye and your 2 physical eyes, form a pyramid – all three should be open and active.

This exercise can help to develop your Mind's Eye.

- Stand or sit and close your eyes.
- Palms facing your body, at upper chest, throat level.

- Very slowly make Figure 8's with your hands in front of you.
- Start at upper chest and move up to your 3rd Eye.
- Do it a couple of times.
- Can you 'see' the movement? (You can probably feel it).
- Your mind's eye will try and tune in and if you can do this you will begin to 'see' from the inside before you see from the outside.

- *Place your fingertips over your 3rd Eye.*
- *Slowly and firmly move your fingers over to the temples to open the 3rd eye.*
- *Repeat several times – slowly. At the same time visualising your 3rd eye opening. Figure 8 over it for a few seconds.*
- *Spin a class crystal prism over it for the reflected light to energise it.*

- Massage a little Frankincense oil or tape resin on your forehead, just above/between the eyebrows[15] to integrate the balance.
- If you are experienced with crystals, choose the crystal of your choice to place on the 3rd eye for a few minutes – you will need to lie down for this. For example: Tiger's Eye. Always energy test to make sure it is supportive to you at this time, especially in the

---

[15] Use your intuition to locate your 3rd Eye – normally located either between the eyebrows or just above them in the centre of the forehead.

case of high frequency crystals such as Herkimer Diamonds.

- If you work with essences – dab a little essence of your choice on a piece of cotton wool and place on the 3rd eye.

The 3rd Eye / pineal gland respond to and are stimulated by light. Shine a light onto the area from a distance of about 4 feet, maybe gently figure 8'ing the torch. If you feel you may be sensitive to torchlight, use the gentler light of a candle.

HEART SPIRALLING

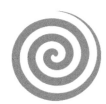 OK, so you are increasing your sensitivity and intuitive 'knowing' – experiment with **spiralling heart energy** to each of the chakras. About 6 inches off the cat's body place your hands above the Heart chakra. This can either be on the chest, if the cat is relaxed or on their back (spine) if they are more relaxed in that position. Either will work as chakra energy goes out the front and back (yin and yang) of the body. Keeping the right hand over the heart, spiral the left hand down to the 3rd chakra (solar plexus) – keep that hold for a few seconds, bringing heart energy to the chakra. Spiral the left hand up to the throat, keep that hold for a few seconds, bringing heart energy to the throat. Spiral to 1st (root) chakra and hold both. Spiral up to crown chakra and hold. Spiral down and

up to 3rd eye. End with both hands over the heart chakra.

Access the torso chakras on the Yin front or the Yang back – see which the animal prefers. The actual chakra energy runs through the body, think of a vortex coming out the front and another out the spine. On humans we tend to work the Yin (front) but often animals feel 'safer' and less anxious when you work the chakras along the spine. The abdominal area is vulnerable and an animal will not expose it unless they feel safe, which is not going to be the case if they feel under threat. To balance a chakra simply circle over it slowly with the palm of your hand for a minute.

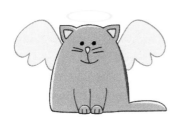

The aura – I have been mentioning it a lot, it is an essential part of animal healing. Do click on this link to see what happens to our auras when we greet our animals...

https://www.youtube.com/watch?v=x1B7lFAmhcs

WORKING WITH THE AURA (also known as the bio-field) has two key benefits:

1. Any disturbance will be felt in the aura before it hits the body, so balancing the aura reduces the risk of that disturbance manifesting as a physical dis-ease. So aura work can be preventative.

2. If you fix something in the physical, work outwards to the aura and fix it in that field too to reduce the risk of the dis-ease returning. Particularly pertinent in cancer.

Dr Valerie Hunt maintained that if you heal the physical body you need to heal the bio field (aura) too to achieve 100% healing and reduce the risk of the dis-ease returning, she specifically mentions Cancer. If you work with the aura of a physically healthy animal you may be able to prevent any energy 'disturbance' from manifesting as a physical dis-ease.

One of the easiest ways of working with an animal is simple 'hands on' **aura sensing; done from the heart with lashings of love**. If you are unfamiliar with this, there is no mystery; here's an easy way to start:

You might like to have done one of the sensitivity exercises mentioned above. Sit quietly with your cat and say a small 'prayer' to ensure that the healing you give will come only from the highest source of love.

You could say something like:

May I bring healing energies of the highest love and light to Mumkin today, in the most divine way.

Lay your hands gently on your cat, anywhere that draws you, or where you know there is a problem, take a couple of deep breaths. Lift your hands off the actual fur and skin and hover over the body about an inch or two away.

A note here, if you are dealing with a nervous or abused animal, introduce your hand from behind so that it does not appear so threatening. You might also like to introduce it with little finger leading, your little finger represents your heart energy and is a very acceptable energy for the cat.

With an abused animal, pay extra attention to working from the heart and with the soul... They will pick it up and feel safer. If you are working with cattle or wild animals do this from a distance – the scanning may be more difficult to do but not impossible, you will just have to focus and concentrate more... After that a domestic cat will seem easy!

You are connecting to her aura: Slowly run your hand 2" – 3" above her body from head to tail, sensing where there is any change of energy in your hands – e.g. hot cold, something pushing/pulling, sluggishness, change of taste in your mouth, unexpected emotions you may feel.

You may sense nothing the first few times you do this, *it doesn't matter,* it's worth persevering – one day you will and – it's a wonderful feeling when you first feel her energy; and once you have, there is no going back, your ability grows. Until then, just *trust* that running your hands over her, scanning her, in this manner will be balancing in some way and a possible catalyst to repair.

When you detect a change, keep your hand over that place until you feel it shift for the positive and then move on. You may feel inclined to trace a small figure 8 or circle your hand, give your intuition free rein. Don't judge it, force it or doubt it.

If there is pain in an area, there is a simple technique, similar to syphoning, **'unwind' the pain out of the body**:

* With your left hand over the painful area, make anti-clockwise circles, connecting to the cat's energy and slowly spiral it out of her, moving your hand further and further away and then shaking the pain off your hand. The energy of pain can sometimes form a 'vortex' over the area and this spiralling of your hand begins to clear it.

* Now place the right hand over the area and circle clockwise over the area – just a dozen times, which will have the effect of stabilising the shift you have just made.

* End by figure 8'ing out to arm length.

Rescan the area and it should feel constant.

If you cannot easily 'feel' the aura, you can surrogate test it: scan and test the surrogate – remember, she's just an extension of your cat's paw. If there is no surrogate available, self-test to detect any tear, hole or rip in the aura and don't forget to re-test after the correction to make sure it worked.

> Use your instinct on how to **end any 'session'**.
> I often gently stroke around the ears, cradle her face
> and kiss her forehead (but that's me, I'm soft and I
> might not choose to do that to a curly-haired pig!).
> As with all work of this kind, thank the 'Universal
> Energy' for any healing that has taken place.

Sometimes healing is not immediately evident – there are no trumpet fanfares or instant miracles but there may be a subtle shift that will result in an improvement in a day or two, or even longer. You may have been a **catalyst to resetting her inner healer**.

A CAT IN THE HAND

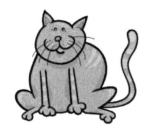

A 'healing' method that is superb if your cat doesn't want to be touched or is away from you, in the veterinary surgery or hospital, is to imagine her the size of a chess piece sitting in your cupped hands in front of your chest (you can also hold a photo or a piece of her fur to help you focus). This is effectively your Heart centre. With your imaginary pet in your hands, send pure love, healing, replenishing energy to that little feline figure, perhaps figure 8'ing between your heart and the figure, to deepen the connection. Smile as you do it and don't doubt the bond of love and its power to support her natural healing abilities.

Always visualise your animal as fit, well and healthy. Manifestation follows thought, so if your cat has a swelling, visualise the swelling subsiding. If she has stiff joints visualise them mobile and flexible.

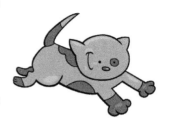

BE NUMERO UNO

Doing any healing work is not advisable if you have taken alcohol, drugs, are under major stress, are really tired or sick yourself. Depression is also an energy that is not conducive to healing. Take care of yourself first. It's a little bit like the safety instructions on a plane: put on your oxygen mask first before you help anyone else. Even as I write this (and I know it to be true), my old conditioning of 'being selfish' raises its annoying little head – many of us have that programming of putting others first. NO!!!!! YOU have to be top of your care list, if you are looking after yourself you will be, long term, far more helpful to your beloved pets, family and friends.

I want you to put the book down for a minute. Sit quietly, close your eyes, stroke the inside of your forearm (doesn't matter what side) and gently say to yourself, while smiling:

It is now safe for me to be Number One on my care list, it is the right thing to do and I do it in the most divine way.
All is well.

This should become a familiar mantra as you repeat it regularly to remind yourself that it's OK to be #1!

If you are balanced and strong by sheer osmosis, without doing anything, you will positively influence your cat's energy and health. So just being with her is good medicine for her.

POLARITY ISSUES

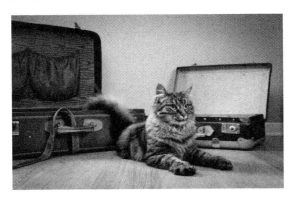

Is your cat a traveller? She could have polarity issues – You cat will have a specific magnetic polarity in her body, as do we humans. Her paws (our feet) are South and seek the North which is represented by the earth we walk upon. So in a healthy cat, as she walks upon the earth there is a definite connection through which she can expel any tired energy and new, refreshing, healing Yin energy will feed her body. She is literally a conduit between heaven and earth.

However, if she is put under any stress, especially related to travelling, which by definition 'unearths' us, be it by car, train or plane. Her polarity can reverse itself and instead of being able to receive this particular source of energy, her body will repel it.

Not ideal and over time and can have an impact, weakening her overall health.

If you suspect this, you can test with a surrogate, simply place the palm of your hand, or your fingertips, over her head and test: it should be strong as the palm and the pads of the fingertips represent South and the top of her head North – so they connect. If it tests weak do a second test, this time put the top of your hand / fingernails (these represent North) on her head and test – if this tests strong it confirms the suspicion that her polarities have reversed.

So to recap:

- Finger pads/palm should be strong
- Finger nails/top of hands should be weak

To return the polarity to default simply spin a cut glass crystal prism ball over her meridian endings. If you don't have a prism simply use a finger (either index or middle will do) place pad on the end of a meridian then quickly flip over and place the nail on it – repeat rapidly for a dozen or so turns. Move onto the next meridian and do the same. Work through all 14 meridians (remember to include Central and Governing).

Retest and the polarity should now have returned to default.

MIR-Method

There is a remarkable woman in the Netherlands, called Mireille Mettes, who has developed a technique called MIR-Method. Mental & Intuitive Reset Method (MIR in Russian means peace). This technique can be adapted for animals and

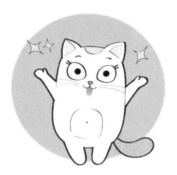

Mumkin adores it. Visit her site for full information and an excellent video where she explains the method clearly and concisely. You can also join her mailing list and get some excellent mailings. She freely shares her wisdom and knowledge, as a gift to the world, although there is a great pdf-book download you can purchase.

http://www.mirmethod.com/

Try it on yourself first and see how it feels and what results you achieve. If you have belief in it, because you will have felt it, then that belief has an energy of its own that empowers the work you subsequently do with your cat.

HOW TO DO IT: It is very simple and only takes you 2 x 2 minutes per day, but important that it is done correctly to optimise the beneficial effects. You are going to relax the body and give short and clear commands. 9 in total that Mireille has identified as being the optimum healing repertoire, by using muscle testing

Instructions: Start stroking circles on the back of one hand, doesn't matter which hand and you can change hands during the procedure. It doesn't even have to be the hand, so long as it is bare skin. It could be the inner arm or even the temples – experiment and see what feels most comforting and relaxing to you. For your cat, if she is relaxed you can do it on her tummy, if not and she is curled up you can do it on her shoulders, base of spine or round the ears.

T Touch® would be a perfect touch technique.

Now say the 9 statements out loud 3 times each while continuing to stroke.

1. Optimise acidity
2. Detox all toxicity
3. Detach father. Detach mother.
4. Clear meridians
5. Supplement all shortages
6. Balance hormone system
7. Fulfill basic needs
8. Optimise chakras and aura
9. Clarify mission

Mireille Mettes has tested and researched this extensively and finds that this is the order the body receives most effectively. The 9 steps must be completed and are connected to each other and work together in a natural synergy.

It takes less than two minutes to do and ideally you should do it twice a day for 4 weeks. You have activated your body, or your cat's, to self-heal and the effect should last 19 months but if you require 'help' before then just go back to it, at any time.

Because it's so soporific and relaxing, your cat should accept the statements – no barriers, they are sensitive to the energy and intent of the words.

With any healing technique you use, Mireille also states that it is important to respect your cat and tell them what you plan to do and literally ask if they are OK with it – if they are not they will probably walk away or, in the case of my cat Mumkin, give me a 'dirty look' – in which case I'll try another technique, if I get the same response to that suggestion I take it

that she probably just wants to be left alone to sleep and relax – I always honour that and never force or overwhelm her with work, however well intentioned.

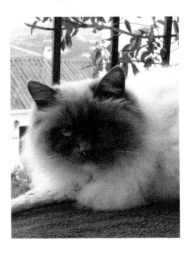

This is Mumkin's 'princess look' – which is basically... *'Don't even think about it!!!'* – Often you will find that when an animal has 'had enough' they will throw you off, you will just have a desire to take your hands away or literally feel the energy pushing you away. Animals are not tactful, you WILL feel it!

The MIR-Method is a **_free_** healing method, as a gift to the world. If you like the sound of it, go to the home page: **www.mirmethod.com** and view the complete **instruction video**. Subscribe to the newsletter and the free 6 weeks' guidance emails for extra support and understanding of the method!

--oOo--

TOUCH

Often by gently touching **with loving intent** you are able to get the animal to feel safe enough so it's body begins to 'listen' to the energies of the healing. **Without doubt, touch can be a springboard to self-healing for the animal**. Observation and sensitivity will make it clear to you what type of touch your cat will prefer.

Linda Tellington-Jones really appreciated this when developing her work which has specific touch techniques that send signals along the nerve pathways, instantly calming the animal and allowing self-healing to take place. I have been a huge fan of her work for decades, all my animals have benefited from her TTouch® and I urge you to take time to explore her site, get on her mailing list for some great information on books and training. This is a truly extraordinary woman and her work has a touch of magic.   http://www.ttouch.com/

THE DIVINE CODES

OK if energy is everything – everything has a frequency. I was assistant to a truly remarkable naturopathic doctor (Michel Burt) and part of his repertoire was Radionics where everything had a

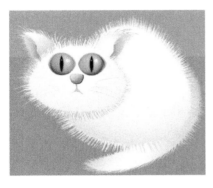 specific vibration and working with those vibrations could help the body heal. I was witness to some astonishing cures. You can use the pure radionics codes but if you are beginning this work with

animals, The Divine Codes will work very well. The divine codes are absolutely 'free' – in fact that is part of their cumulative energy – they are not sold.

They can be found on:

http://reikidoc.blogspot.com.es/2014/06/divine-healing-codes-and-how-to-use-them.html

I have embedded those relevant to animals here for your convenience but the whole philosophy of these codes is that they are freely available to everyone.

You can test to see if they strengthen your cat. So for example, she has a wound – energy test with a surrogate over the site of the wound and it will probably test weak, which confirms there is a problem with the area. Write the Divine code either in the air above the wound or on a piece of paper and hold it in the air over the wound.

The spaces between the numbers are IMPORTANT– be sure to copy them exactly as written for them to work.

Leave for ten seconds and energy test again – strong? Then the frequency of the code is helping and supporting the pet's own self-healing mechanism. Still weak? Then try another code or something else. The body will guide you to what it needs. There is no one model that has the answer for all cats at all times.

For Animals

- 29 56 7892156   for abused animals
- 29 58 734   for wound care for animals
- 21 76 9654321   for animals who suffer from malnutrition
- 86 55 158   for the wild animals to have their habitat increase
- 33 37 899   (human code is safe for animals) for removal of parasites, worms, and also etheric attachments / parasites
- 96 76 269   for ear fungus and mites
- 42 92 532   for dry skin itching
- 81 50 561   for skin sensitivity from friction and loss of fur or hair

For Felines

- 21 76 582   for assisting with hair balls
- 92 72 821   for feline lower urinary tract infection
- 51 28 765   for feline eye problems

If you are not sure TEST TEST TEST. It will guide you in the right healing direction for the animal.

Testing has many uses, let's look at how you would use it to test a divine code on a wound. Point to the wound on the animal, focus on it, make the statement you are testing the wound and energy test your quads... it should test weak as the wound will be causing a disturbance in the energies. Now put the divine code in the air above the wound, hold it there for ten seconds and energy test with intention... If the divine code is going to be helpful in the healing process it will test strong, if not try another one and if you can't find a healing code that is appropriate, try something else (see the guidance grid at the end of the book).

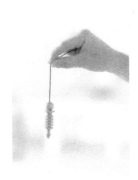

Pendulums are the most popular dowsing instruments. Lightweight and portable a pendulum can slip into your pocket wherever you go.

A useful tool for a healthier lifestyle. A pendulum is a bridge between your rational and intuitive minds. It allows you to access the WISE ONE WITHIN.

We all know exactly what we need to optimise our health or the health of our feline friends, but that knowledge sometimes gets lost through the demands of contemporary life and the lack of validation as we grow up. After you have been using the pendulum for a while, you will begin to observe that your natural instinct and intuition becomes stronger.

Dowsing is still used in some Mediterranean countries to find water; in rural areas especially of France and Spain, the Water Dowser is part of the community. There are different types of dowsing, you will find the one that you are best at. Some people are great at health issues but cannot find water or vice versa.

What is it? A simple weight on a thread – that weight may be a cotton reel or a solid gold pendant, large or small, light or heavy, simple or ornate – it is entirely your choice, a ring on the thread, even a teabag on a string will work.

Length of thread: you will need enough to permit movement. A long thread produces a slow, lazy movement that takes its time changing. A shorter thread produces a faster movement.

Prepare yourself: 3 thumps, hook up. Get yourself tuned in.

Nobody really knows how or why dowsing works, it just seems to. Let go of your left brain and it's rational thoughts and open the door to your more intuitive right brain.

Garbage in, garbage out. As with energy testing, success is dependent on an open mind asking the right question. If you don't ask the right question you will not get the right answer.

Know what you are asking. "Is Mumkin OK?" is a bit too vague, what do I mean? Whereas – "is this divine code the optimum treatment for Mumkin's wound right now?" is more precise and focussed so the response will be more precise.

Dowsing answers through our subconscious and sometimes, our subconscious wants to please us, so it will give us the answer we want to hear. For example: Does Mumkin have Cancer? I guarantee it will swing 'no' unless you are able to truly centre and detach yourself emotionally from the question. Know your boundaries and define the extent of the job you are asking a pendulum to do.

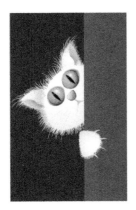

One way to stop your subjective desire for an answer is to keep asking:

"I wonder what the answer will be? Whatever it is I have a choice, but it would be good to know the truth. That is what I seek – THE TRUTH. And what I do with that is up to me"

Basic holding: when you start, follow these instructions and as you gain confidence you can change any aspect of them to suit your personal style as you discover what works best for you. The elbow should be below the shoulder and the wrist below the elbow. Hold the thread between the thumb and index finger, both pointing down.

Make sure your hands or legs are not crossed or touching each other. Sit with feet apart and firmly planted on the ground.

If you are right handed use your right hand and if left handed use your left.

The start position: hold the pendulum and ask: *show me my start position* – see how it responds, it might not move at all. There is no universally, correct, response. My personal one is back and forth. I also call it my 'idiot swing'.

It is a good idea to keep the pendulum moving in a gentle to and fro swing, think of it like a neutral swing.

Defining the swings:

Show me 'yes' – relax and see how it swings

Show me 'no' – relax and see how it swings

Double check by asking:

Is my name Minnie Mouse? – observe swing

Is my name ....?   – observe swing

You are communicating with your subconscious and setting up a code, defining a language. It takes time for clear communication to develop, so make a commitment to practise daily to lay a firm foundation for your future dowsing.

Hold your pendulum in the start position and ask:

Show me my 'maybe'/wrong question swing

Observe how it swings

You now have 4 swings to choose from:

Start position
Yes
No
Maybe /wrong question

3 key questions to ask in preparation:

CAN I?
MAY I?
AM I READY?

Can I? – This is asking if your dowsing skills are developed enough or the task in hand. You may be able to dowse to see if a carrot is good for you, but not yet able to find the lost key ring.

May I? – This is asking permission. It is wise to seek permission in healing work, especially with cats as they can be very discerning and discriminating in their personal energy.

Am I ready? – Is there something else you need to do to prepare for the dowsing (e.g. get more centred).

If you proceed against any of these three questions, you cannot trust the answers.

WE CAN USE IT WITH OUR ANIMALS TO GET STRAIGHTFORWARD ANSWERS – *Is this the optimum treatment for Mumkin's injury now?*

It will be a useful aid to point you in the right direction... After all there are many ways up the same healing mountainside and you just want to pick the most effective for your animal at this moment in time; that is why I developed the Guidance Grid (later in the book) to help guide you through the labyrinth.

We can also use it to measure the energy of your animal's chakras – you do not ask any question, it tells you how strong the energy flows are. Hold it over the chakra and observe how it spins. The stronger and faster the spin the stronger the chakra.

A practical experiment – why not dowse for the optimum colour of bedding for your animal and then the optimum position for its bed.

Animals are sensitive to GEOPATHIC STRESS and a simple thing like moving their bed can help their energy stabilise.

Interestingly **cats are attracted to areas where energy is high**. Be careful they don't absorb too much negative energy. I had a cat who used to sit outside my treatment room door, he wanted to help everyone that came to me. In the end I had to remove him to another part of the house because I could see he was helping by absorbing negativity BUT at too high a cost to himself. I remember Donna Eden told me he had a unique aura (she sees energy) that she had never seen on an animal before and Boris's energy held NO fear, only love and healing... He really was a 'master healer'. But I still had to make sure he didn't *OVER*do it.

On the other end of the scale, horses, dogs, birds and pigs will **avoid negative or disturbed energy**; they love harmony and a smooth energy flow. If you are a horse lover, you will probably have observed this.

Common sense tells us not to put their beds near **electrical appliances** and not to use **toxic cleaning agents** near them. Make sure their food and drinking bowls are not toxic plastic.

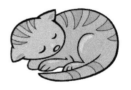

For those of you familiar with Dr Emoto's work. He found that two of the most powerfully healing words, in any language, are LOVE and GRATITUDE... Write these words on a piece of paper and pop under your cat's food and water bowls – it enhances the vibrational quality of the food and drink.

DIET

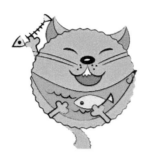

Obviously diet impacts on your cat's health. Energy testing (preferably with a surrogate) food and drinks, can be immensely useful in fine-tuning your cat's diet to suit her body chemistry and needs.

You may be surprised – expensive products are not necessarily the best for your cat – it's what suits her chemistry at this precise moment in time. Many years ago I held a pet workshop and bought every conceivable dog food you could get your hands on – we tested them 'blind' and it was interesting that some of the cheaper brands suited the dogs very well and some of the more expensive 'organic' brands didn't. That's not to say there was anything wrong with them, they just didn't suit the pet's chemical make-up.

Surrogate test everything she eats and the water she drinks. If you don't have a surrogate available, self-test or use the pendulum. If anything tests weak, eliminate it from her diet for ten days and she how she reacts. This is particularly useful when animals **have skin, or even behavioural/aggression problems.**

The test is simple – hold a sample of the food against her (normally against her spine) and energy test the surrogate or yourself. No need to ask questions, you are simply testing how her body reacts when you introduce the substance into her field.

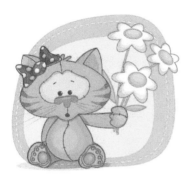

If you work with them, energy test **flower essences** – this will give you a clue as to the emotional state of the animal and a few drops in their water – or on your hands as you stroke them – can help recalibrate emotions.

Ideally animals should not be taken away from their mother before 8 weeks. If you are in a position that you have a young animal under 8 weeks, handle and give it love every day, get friends to come and do the same so it feels, loved, accepted and unconcerned by different energies in the new mixed species 'litter'.

When the problem is emotional, flower essences are easy, safe and effective, in fact animals can respond more quickly to them than humans do. They will support, on an emotional level, any treatment your cat is receiving or help her through an emotional upset (e.g. firework night or separation anxiety).

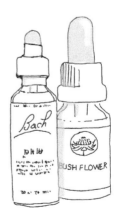

There are now myriad essences available. My two personal favourites are:

- ❧ The Australian Bush Flower Remedies[16]
    - ❧ Healing Herbs[17]

There is nothing new about these flower essences. Flowers and plants have been used since the beginning of time by healers of all cultures. Every flower and plant has a specific vibrational energy that can influence your cat in a subtle, safe and positive way.

These essences capture that energy in a 'homeopathic' liquid form. The plant or flower is picked at dawn (the zenith of their vitality) and placed in water, in the sunlight, for several hours. The liquid is then strained and forms the base of the essence. It has no actual molecules of the plant or flower and as such not to be confused with herbal tinctures.

Adding a few drops to your cat's drinking water will begin to balance out her emotions and energy. 3 drops in a normal cat bowl should be enough. Be reassured that they are <u>self-adjusting</u> and as such whatever dose you administer, no harm will come to your cat. Very occasionally, there may be a mini 'healing crisis' as emotions come to the surface, but this should pass very quickly (within 24 hours).

---

[16] www.ausflowers.com.au

[17] www.healingherbs.co.uk this is a company that backs Dr Bach remedies in the 'old-fashioned' way and to a high quality.

If your cat turns up her nose at the water – rub the drops into your hand instead and stroke over her aura. It's not quite as good as drinking the essence, but the vibrational quality is still shared.

You can use a surrogate to test which flower essence is needed. Simply hold the essence against the cat's body and test the surrogate (who will be connected via her other hand to your cat).

* If the test is weak, then don't use it.

* If the test is strong then it could either be 'neutral' or strengthening to your cat. To determine which:

* Weaken the cat (or surrogate) by tracing down from mouth to pelvic area. Repeat the test.

* If it's weak then the essence is neutral, it won't do any harm but neither will it strengthen your cat. It's a signal to seek another essence or route up the mountainside of healing.

* However if it now tests strong then voila! It has the power to strengthen that weak muscle and is therefore going to have a positive impact on your cat.

Keep your feet on the ground and objectively evaluate your cat's behaviour and health over the next couple of weeks. Observe and see if there is an improvement or subtle shift. Don't fall foul to ENCS *(Emperor's New Clothing Syndrome)* – stay objectively discerning.

If you don't have any essences you can download the lists. Put your finger onto each individual essence available and energy test the statement:

IS THIS THE OPTIMUM ESSENCE TO USE NOW TO HELP MUMKIN'S WOUND HEAL?

The essence that is the 'odd man out' will be the essence you can then purchase for your cat.

Essences can be obtained easily online nowadays either direct or from one of my favourite sites www.nutricentre.com

If you feel your cat is responding well, you might like to research in more depth with either of these companies.

www.healingherbs.co.uk – I choose this company because it was started by a single person in 1988 who wanted to keep it small and prepare the essences with total integrity. Julian Barnard is still involved in every step of the process. If you would like more details about Dr Bach and the remedies, there is an educational section on the site with many free videos, he has been very generous with his information.

www.ausflowers.com.au – is the main site with distributors in the UK. Ian White set up ABFE and has also kept his hand firmly on the rudder. I find they nearly always test strong on clients – find the right one and they really make a difference.

Here are a few that might interest you:

The essences in *italics* are Australian Bush and in normal typeface are Healing Herbs.

Black Eyed Susan	*Is THE stress and anxiety essence for cats. Also good for irritability.*	*Sundew*	*To help your cat focus*
Chicory	For the cat who is always seeking attention and is unhappy being left alone.	Walnut or *Bottlebrush*	To help her cope with change. So great for if you are moving house.
Dog Rose	*For the fearful or shy cat.*	*Flannel Flower*	*For the cat that doesn't like to be touched. Try some before grooming or a massage.*
Holly *Mountain Devil*	*For a suspicious cat that does not trust.* *For cats who have suffered past abuse. Especially good if you are trying to introduce a second cat into the home. Or if the owner is having a baby.*	Aspen	*For a nervous kitten or cat especially in unfamiliar surroundings.*
Impatiens	For the impatient, irritable kitty.	Chestnut	Helps break bad habits.

Mimulus	For the cat who is always fearful of the slightest sound or movement. This is the one to use when you KNOW what she is afraid of, e.g. fireworks.	Honeysuckle	If you suspect your cat will miss you while she is in the cattery. Or if you are inheriting an animal from someone who has had to move on.
Star of Bethlehem	Perfect for rescue cats. Trauma, grief, injury or abuse.	Vervain Or Crowea	Will calm down a hyped up, over stressed cat.
Gymea Lily	Posture, aching bones, spinal alignment	Olive	For the exhausted cat.

And of course, the classic Dr Bach Rescue Remedy, 5 Flowers or the ABFE Emergency Essence are all essentials in a time of trauma or shock. Try them out next November 5th – Guy Fawkes Night. Begin administering a couple of hours before the fireworks are due to start.

http://ausflowers.com.au/Products/Single-Essences
link for the single essences.

HOMEOPATHY

I'm a huge fan of **homeopathy** and ARNICA is my trusted friend. I'm very excited to have discovered Madeleine Innocent – here are links to her website and also the training, should you be interested. You may not intend to become a homeopath but might like a little more information on how to use homeopathy with you animals (and on yourself too).

http://twolegsandfour.com/opal.html
            - this is the training

http://twolegsandfour.com/
                - this is her general website and blog

You can energy test homeopathic remedies (in the same way as flower essences) to identify the optimum for this moment in time for a particular problem. I always energy test and trust it 100% BUT it's also good to have a little knowledge to enhance that trust.

TALK FROM THE HEART and the cells listen.

Talking, either in your head or out loud, from the heart, with loving intent to your cat WILL have an effect. You need to be grounded and balanced first, so that a clear channel is created, **by osmosis** you can affect an animal before you even start talking. If your energies are balanced and grounded it can jump-start theirs onto the path to harmony. Think of yourself as a human jump lead.

The secret to communicating with your animal is to be still and open and trust what comes into your mind's eye or ear. Animals will often find it easier to **communicate with images**.

You may hear words, you may see pictures, you may suddenly just have a 'knowing' or you may feel sensations in your body that reflect the animal's feelings.

The secret is the open mind, however bizarre the images that come into it, don't dismiss them as 'poppycock' – take a moment to think of their possible associations, you may be surprised at the message you receive and how accurate it is.

If you did this every day with your animal, over time you would become VERY good at 'getting' the message!

You might consider writing down what you 'receive', it's very easy to forget it.

Try asking a simple question: ***How can I help you?*** And see what response you get.

My friend Anne Wilson, the animal communicator, once told me that one of my cats insisted that she tell me that I was to stop serving her food out of that 'cold box in the corner' (i.e. the fridge) – sometimes it's such a small thing that can make a big difference.

YOUR CAT'S BODY IS LISTENING.

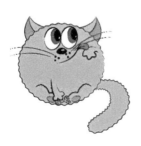

Don't doubt that your body, and your cat's, has its own consciousness, every single part of it and that consciousness responds to your thoughts and words. They can be good energy medicine or seriously hinder your body's health and well-being.

Your body can hear you and your cat's body can hear you, so take advantage of that wonderful ability and talk positive, with compassion and love. Over time the conversations will get easier. I know this may sound strange now, especially if you are not used to working with energy, but it is a natural, organic process and is totally safe to explore.

Dr Cleve Backster spent 36 years researching bio-communication in plant, animal and human cells. He identified key factors in this concept: real intent, attunement and spontaneity of emotions (i.e. true not forced emotions). The emotions can elicit an electrical reaction in the cells.

And finally, when your cat is feeling a little under the weather, here's something to help you decide what might be the most appropriate technique to use.

MADDIE'S GUIDANCE GRID

To help give you direction
when 'intuition' is thin on the ground:

WHAT IS THE PRIORITY/OPTIMUM
TREATMENT TO WORK WITH TODAY TO...

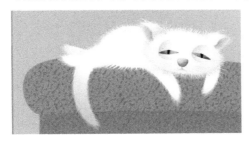

(here add something specific to your cat e.g. heal the wound on Mumkin's paw).

Fill in the grid below with all the techniques you feel resonate with you – it can be half a dozen or all of them from this little book, along with other 'common-sense' or modalities you might be qualified in or heard about. Make up another page if you need it – my grid runs into several. You can then energy test to see what is the PRIORITY for the animal right now. Everything will probably have some positive benefit on the animal, but this helps you discover the MOST EFFECTIVE road to healing.

So with your question clearly in your mind (see above) you say:

Is it in Column A? – test each column until you find an odd one out, so you know that the optimum treatment, the priority at this moment in time is in that particular column.

Now test each box in the column (*Is this the priority treatment?*) until you find the odd one out – THIS is what will benefit your cat today.

A	B	C	D	E

WALKING THE TIGHTROPE

*A state of balance is very rarely a truly static state for a
human being or any animal. Harmony is like walking a
tightrope; we constantly have to move
and compensate to maintain our balance.
It's a natural dance to be enjoyed and mastered.*

I have talked in the book about getting balanced
before working on your cat. What do I mean by that?
Basically, before working with energy you want to
make sure your own in running the right direction, is
crossing as it should and is not chaotic or 'scrambled'
– it need only take a few seconds, but get into the
habit of balancing yourself first, it will make all the
difference to the quality and effectiveness of your
treatments.

The basic balancing techniques are:

* FOUR 'THUMPS'
* CROSS CRAWL
* TIBETAN MEDITATION POSE
* HOOK UP

Form your thumb and first two fingers into a triad and

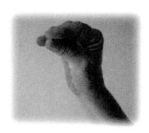

firmly massage or tap the
points described below.

If you have long nails, simply
improvise and use your
knuckles. Don't forget to
breathe and smile while you
tap.

The first 'thump' is K27

The benefits of this simple exercise include:

* 'Flips' energy into forward flow.
* Jump-starts and energises the entire system.
* Balances disruptions caused by travelling, especially through time zones. (A great one to do during a flight and when you step off the plane.)
* Brings clarity to thought.
* Improves focus and concentration.
* Brings a flow back into your life.
* Temporarily energises the eyes, useful if you are tired but still have a few more miles to drive.

You will be tapping and therefore stimulating the 27th acupuncture point on each Kidney meridian. These important points act as 'junction boxes' for other meridians.

They are located near the 'right angle' where the collar and breast bones meet. You will feel two natural

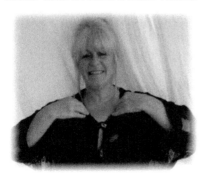

indentations that may be slightly tender when you press them.

Don't worry if you can't find the exact points, you know the approximate area, so tap around and you will get them, as with all energy work, it is about intention and attention.

Breathe, fully moving your ribcage and diaphragm.

Smile and tap for 5 seconds... YES, that's all it takes.

THE TARZAN THUMP!

Benefits of this second thump include:

- ❧ Stimulates the Thymus gland.
- ❧ Supports the Immune System.
- ❧ Helps cope with the body's stress response and negative emotional energies.
- ❧ Stimulates overall energy and vitality – primates will thump this gland to increase their strength before mating or fighting.
- ❧ Places the body in a temporary state of 'balance'.

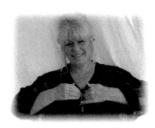

You will be tapping over the Thymus Gland[18] which is located in the middle of your chest – exactly where Tarzan thumps, in fact rather than tapping; you could clench your fists and thump your chest like Tarzan!

Breathe, smile and tap/thump for 5 seconds.

---

[18] The Australian psychiatrist, Dr John Diamond (*Your Body Doesn't Lie*) www.drjohndiamond.com - made a study of the Thymus gland and suggests we 'waltz' the thymus, i.e. tap lightly to the waltz rhythm ... 123 123 123, smile and look at something beautiful while you are tapping to increase the effectiveness of the exercise.

THE MONKEY THUMP

Benefits of monkey thumping include:

* Boosts Immune System and general energy levels.

* Increases your ability to accept/metabolise changes.

* Balances blood chemistry.

* Aids detoxification of the body.

* Helps metabolise and absorb nutrients.

* Improves absorption of supplements (tap for a few seconds before and after taking them).

You will be massaging/tapping/thumping the 21st acupressure points on each Spleen meridian. These 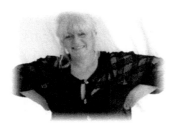 are located on the side of the ribcage, roughly where the bottom line of a bra would sit (see photo). You will know when you hit on them as they will be tender.

Once located, use your clenched fists to massage, tap or thump firmly the points for a minimum of 5 seconds. Breathe and smile.

You can also work on the Spleen lymphatic points: simply lean back slightly, opening up the ribcage and tap round from Sp21 to underneath each breast in line with the nipples.

Cheeky thump

* Relieves anxiety.

* Helps you begin to trust in the mystery of life.

* Helps in letting issues pass through, be digested and released.

* Balanced Stomach energy encourages you to pay attention to self-care.

* Helps achieve a clear thought process.

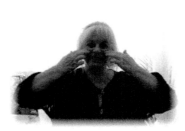

Called the 'Great Bone Hole' they are located slightly below the apex of your cheeks when you smile, in line with your eye and the edge of your nostril.

Again, do for 5 seconds.

Thymus pressure with prayer

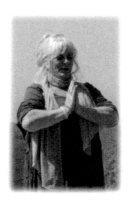

Place your palms together in a prayer position. Forearms parallel with the floor. Thumbs will be over the Thymus gland, push against this point firmly for ten seconds then release. Repeat. This brings you into a temporary state of balance and in the ancient Indian tradition, connects you to your soul.

Say a simple thank you for all your blessings, one of which is your 4-legged friend.

CROSS CRAWL – 20 seconds

The body functions with crossing patterns, curves, roundness and above all, flow. There are very few sharp edges in the human body.

This technique is based on the fact that the left hemisphere of the brain needs to send information to the right side of the body and the right hemisphere to the left side. If either of these 'communication tracts' are not adequately flowing and open then it will be impossible to access the brain's full capacity or the body's full intelligence.

The bottom line is: when our energies are crossed every system in the body and the body's healing abilities is encouraged to optimum efficiency, we are literally healthier. However, when the energies are not crossed, the healing abilities are dramatically reduced.

We are born with the energies running in a parallel pattern, homolaterally[19] down the body but when, as babies, we start to crawl; the crossover pattern and left/right brain integration really begins to take form. This is why children who do not crawl enough can develop learning difficulties. So don't just plonk your baby/grandchild in a bouncer, let it roam wild – the crawling action will enable enhanced brain function.

---

[19] We use the word homolateral to indicate this parallel patterning. II

Back to us as adults: Nature intended that we cross crawl naturally during the course of each day: walking, running, swimming are all natural ways of consolidating that crossing pattern. However, contemporary lifestyles are increasingly sedentary. In addition, fashion footwear can prohibit good posture and, we carry heavy shoulder bags, briefcases or shopping bags which all inhibit the natural flow of the movement.

Needless to say any stress or trauma in our life can throw the pattern back into homolateral. Our body will give us hints when this happens – for example stop reading right now and see if any 'body part' is crossed – wrists, arms, ankles, legs? This is a message that the body needs / wants to cross its energies, it yearns to run at full efficiency, it seeks balance to do so.

Body language specialists say crossed arms mean a closed off/ defensive stance, but in reality, from an energetic standpoint, it can also mean that you are trying to cross the energies, albeit unconsciously, so that you can truly understand what is being said to you.

So, to summarise; doing a CROSS CRAWL can improve left and right brain integration and encourage energies to cross.

This in turn can:

Greatly improve the body's natural healing ability.

* Enhance the absorption of vitamin supplementation.

- Relieve fatigue, exhaustion and lack of motivation.
- Bring clarity to your thinking.
- Help your whole system function more efficiently.
- Improve co-ordination.
- Reduce certain learning difficulties.
- Stimulate memory.
- Pump lymphatic and cerebrospinal fluid.
- Help you feel more balanced, motivated and energised.
- Harmonise energies and increase natural self healing abilities.
- Ease depression.
- Support the immune system.
- Support and help make more effective any other treatments you may be receiving from your healthcare practitioner.

It is marching on the spot to reprogramme the body into a health supporting crossing pattern, without which you will never heal 100%.

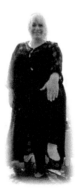

Lift your right arm and right leg together. Then lift your left arm and left leg together. Do you remember the Thunderbird puppets! Repeat a few times/15 seconds or so. This reflects the homolateral, parallel patterning which your brain will recognise and feel

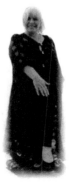

comfortable with if your energies are not crossing.

Now lift your right arm and left leg together (see photo on the right above) followed by left arm and right leg. i.e. diagonal/opposites together. Repeat a few times/15 seconds. This represents the cross over pattern and may feel uncomfortable until your energies reprogramme themselves into a crossing pattern.

Repeat.

ALWAYS end on the cross over pattern and do a few extra 'crosses' to integrate the reprogramming.

To be honest, I don't always feel like doing the full exercise and do this shorter version which I love – and so do my energies:

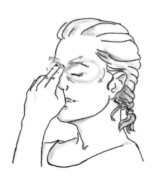

Place your middle finger on your 3rd eye and focus inwards. Slowly and firmly circle round one eye back to 3rd eye and circle round the other eye – this of the 'mask of Zorro'. Do this two or three times and then change direction. Ending with finger on 3rd Eye. Smile and bring your right hand round the left side of your neck, dig in your fingers and pull round to the front of the shoulder and then down diagonally over the torso to the right hip and down and off the right left. Repeat on the other side. Do two or three times. End with both hands over your heart. Smile and say a gentle 'thank you'. Stand tall and take a second to see how you feel – has it made a difference?

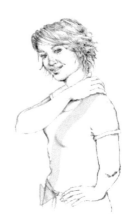

Unscrambling energy – Tibetan meditation pose

This unscrambles the energies making for clearer communication, clearer thinking, improved left/right brain integration and cheers you up in no time at all, so great for when you are feeling sad, confused or angry. It returns your energy circuits to default, reduces stress, and encourages release of past emotional baggage or trauma.

We tend to naturally sit in this position and it may be familiar to you. It is sometimes considered to be a blocking pose but in reality, if you are over-stimulated, you are naturally trying to unscramble so that you can understand more clearly, so it is the total opposite of being blocked, it is about wanting to be open and understanding.

* Sit (or stand), cross the arms over the chest with hands under the armpits, thumbs out and up.
* Close your eyes, breathe and smile.
* Stay in this position until you feel calm.
* Bring your hands into prayer position and take a couple of breaths.

- Put your arms out in front of you, palms facing outwards. Feet are still crossed.

- Cross the wrists and intertwine your fingers, pull them towards you, up and under, so your clasped hands are sitting under your chin. Did you do this when you were a child? I have asked many people from different countries and most have – as children we instinctively get ourselves into positions that encourage balance.

- Close your eyes, breathe and smile. Hold for as long as you want – a minute?

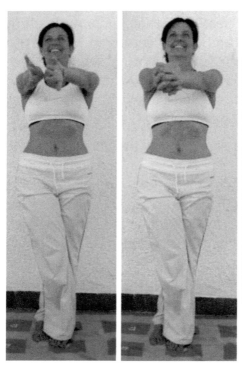
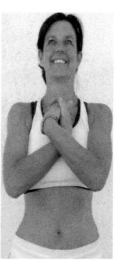

Hook up – a hyperlink to harmony

'Discombobulated' ... I simply love the sound of this word although I have my doubts as to its 'official' existence, but just the sound of it manages to describe how we can all feel occasionally: Uncoordinated in both body and mind; a bit 'off'; a little 'spaced out'; stuck; not fully in the flow of life and unable to cope with the challenges life sets us.

This simple technique is a hyperlink to harmony, equilibrium and balance. It:

* connects (hooks up) two important channels of energies: Governing and Central, which in turn boosts confidence and courage.

* brings clarity of thought and purpose.

* strengthens the auric field, keeping it solid and protective.

* bridges the energies between the head and the body.

* enables you to feel more connected, co-ordinated, grounded and able to cope.

* stimulates the ancient Strangeflow energies.

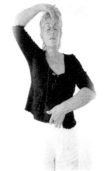

Place the middle finger of one hand on your forehead between the eyebrows, over the 3rd Eye.

Place the middle finger of the other hand in your navel.

With a slight pull of the skin upward on both points, close your eyes, take a deep breath and relax. (Breathe in through the nose and out through the mouth.)

Stay in this position for about twenty seconds (or for however long feels right to you).

By strengthening the Governing Channel that runs up the back, you affect the spine, not only in a physical sense but also in an emotional way – literally giving you the 'backbone' to face and resolve problems and move forward in your life.

By strengthening the Central Channel that runs up the front of the torso you will be less vulnerable to absorbing other people's negative energies. An overdose of these can cause exhaustion and even depression.

It is a powerful tool for quickly centring yourself and has immediate neurological consequences. It has been reported to be helpful to a person starting to seizure.

Try it right now and see if you feel less discombobulated!

If you feel uncomfortable putting your finger in your navel, put it just below your navel, it will still hook up.

HOW TO ENERGY TEST

I am also adding a little bit more information on how to do a basic energy test; beginners among you might find it useful. Get confident testing the person first and then move on to using them as a surrogate.

Energy testing enables us to access the body in a language that is easy to understand.

The body can reveal to us, via the test of applying and resisting pressure on the muscle, if something strengthens or weakens it.

It is truly that simple.

Of course, nuances have been developed and it has become and 'art and science' but never forget, it is simple, easy, organic, safe and with a little practice – accurate.

Please believe me when I say, that with a little practice, anyone and everyone can do these tests. I am <u>not</u> special; it is neither magic nor trickery. It is a **practical bio-feedback tool** to help you tune in to your body's needs. Use it with confidence on your children, spouse and friends.

A few preliminaries…

Spend a minute of getting your basic energies balanced (see above).

Make sure they have **no injuries** or problems that might get in the way of the test. Obviously avoid testing a muscle that is injured or weak for any reason. An accurate result will not be achieved from a shoulder that was dislocated last month!

Neither of you should view this as a **competition** of strength.

It is also not about 'failure' or 'success' – simply discovering the truth so that we can determine the best way forward for your cat.

Check their **posture** is relaxed yet standing straight and nothing is crossed.

Remind them that **BREATHING** normally is essential throughout – do not hold your breath.

Don't try and second guess the test. Be **objective** and ready to embrace the truth!

Common sense dictates that the tests will not be accurate if you have taken recreational **drugs or alcohol**!

Dehydration can affect the test so both of you drink a glass of water beforehand.[20]

Remove any **jewellery** that may get in the way, watch, bangles etc. IF you think about it, sometimes they do not present a problem. My personal rule of thumb is if I think I about it, I remove it.

Don't energy test right next to a computer or electrical equipment.

Testing is very much of the moment, a present tense. It is not a response of yesterday or tomorrow but very much on now, today. Reflect that in your thinking. Bring all your attention to what you are doing. Very easy with an animal because they live so much in the present moment.

---

[20] The test for dehydration is simply to tug at a lock of hair and energy test (ET) if it is weak then dehydration could be an issue.

So, put all expectations aside - take a deep breath and get started. Enjoy and relax into it – I was one of Donna's worst students at first because I SO wanted to be the best (let's not even begin to analyse that!). Once I let go, stopped judging myself and relaxed, hey presto – it worked a dream.

GENERAL INDICATOR MUSCLE

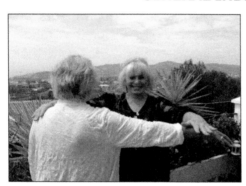

(*Pectoralis Major Clavicular – the smart name for the shoulder muscle which is the one you are isolating and testing.*)

Your friend stands up straight, unclenched fists and relaxed, with feet apart. (If necessary, the test can be done sitting.)

Left arm (or right) is held out at a right angle to the body and parallel to the floor – you have a range to play with here, from straight out to the side or slightly towards midline, experiment to see what feels right to you.

Check hand is *not* clenched into a fist – fingers should be straight.

Stand in front of your friend, not too close, with your right hand, palm flat and facing downwards and fingers extended – resting on your friend's raised arm, on the forearm just near the wrist joint. (Shoulder side of the wrist.) If you test on the other side of the wrist, just the hand will go down not the arm.

The left hand can rest gently on her shoulder to create a full circuit between the two of you.

Demonstrate the range of movement – so that she is confident in what is about to happen. *You are interested in the first couple of inches* of that range, not everyone's arm drops all the way down to their hip. It might be that a 'spongy' response is all that is felt, but that is enough to indicate a weak result.

Tell her to 'HOLD' – wait half a second, while her brain registers the command and then apply pressure for 2 seconds – gently, no jerking movements.

Do not put too much pressure on the arm – the lighter the pressure the better the testing and the less tiring it is for both of you. This becomes particularly relevant when you are doing multiple tests. I often ask students to 'lighten up' even more, they often think it won't work – but it does.

What happened?   If it stays in position easily it means that it is testing STRONG.

However, if it is spongy, or falls all the way down then that is a WEAK test.

To get a feel for what is their personal 'yes' and 'no' – try this:

Get them to say the statement 'my name is Minnie Mouse' (without smiling) – energy test – it should be weak, it is a false statement. They could say anything that is false, e.g. 'my name is Fred, I am standing on the North Pole' – anything that is obviously false. Now do the same with a positive statement such as: 'my name is xxyyzzxx' – should be strong.

When you are both balanced and you are confident in the basic energy test, then simply place the surrogate's hand on the cat and test.

I am posting instruction videos on the Madison's Medicine Facebook page and also on www.midlifegoddess.ning.com but if you have any questions at all, just email me – I'm happy to help clarify anything that is confusing you.

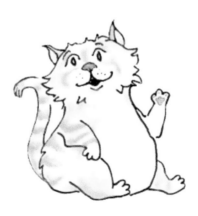

All profits from this book will go to Caroline Cares an animal help and rescue group founded in honour of the wonderful Caroline Walsh who sadly lost her battle with cancer May 2015.

If you would like to make a donation, please visit the Facebook page where the website and donation facility will be shared once available.

https://www.facebook.com/Caroline-Cares-Animal-Rescue-1653643551557292/?fref=ts
(link to Facebook page)

To help promote the book, it would be fantastic if you could take five minutes and write a rave review on the Amazon site – thank you!

I will be posting short video clips on my Facebook page to illustrate some of the techniques. If you find it useful to 'look at' rather than read a technique, connect to:

https://www.facebook.com/Madisons-Medicine-287253251377558/

Or join my closed site – www.midlifegoddess.ning.com

Why did I write this book and who am I?

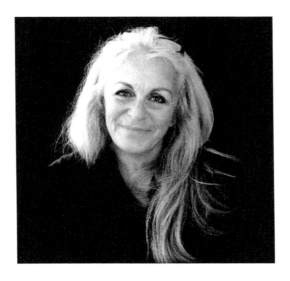

Well I ask myself the latter a lot! Seriously, I wrote this book because working with energy is such an integral part of my life, it naturally spills over into that of my animals. By osmosis they get energy medicine. It seems to me to be a natural progression from stroking your cat to stroking or circling in a specific way that encourages the flow of energy in her body.

I hope this little book will motivate you to experiment with your cat and see which techniques you, and her, enjoy the most. They will then simply weave themselves into your lives, enhancing the already strong bond between the two of you and of course, her health and happiness. Have fun with this, it is nearly all instinctive and a lot you will be doing already.

And me?

Many moons ago I was involved in the heart of London advertising, becoming a successful international board director. However, I realised, after a few ambition fuelled years, that I wanted my life to take a different direction and shocked everyone by giving up the BMW, Armani suits and Gucci briefcase, becoming a student again.

I've trained in massage, sports massage, aromatherapy, Indian head massage, reflexology, trager, nutrition, flower essences, radionics... A true workshop groupie, I proudly filled a wall with qualifications but could not find what I had been seeking; I couldn't even really define it ...until, through divine synchronicity, I met Donna Eden in London through a mutual friend. Within no time at all (6 days to be precise), I was in Ashland in Donna's backyard with about four other students, eagerly learning about energy – this was more than two decades ago, so no information highway was available and ever the thirsty student, I drank in everything I could on these visits, rushing back to London to experiment on my long-suffering clients!

Over the years I crossed the ocean many times learning from Donna and also John Thie (*Touch for Health*).

I then began to teach Donna's work in many parts of the world. I now divide my time between the Isle of Wight and Andalucía and set up and run the Eden Energy Medicine official training in Europe. It's come a long way since those days in her back yard!

If you are interested in extending your energy medicine 'toolkit for health' to the human body, Madison holds workshops in Europe and also a well-established online 'global' study group – MEET@home (Maddie's Essential Everyday Techniques). There is also a weekly 'Bitesize' club. Both are supported by their own 'closed' Facebook pages where you can network with like-minded souls.

Madison can be contacted on:

madisonking@hotmail.com

www.madisonking.com

www.midlifegoddess.ning.com

Facebook: Madison's Medicine (and others)

Other books by Madison – available in print or Kindle download from Amazon, include:

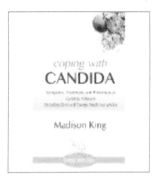
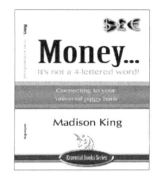

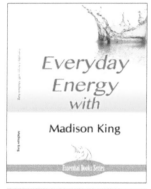
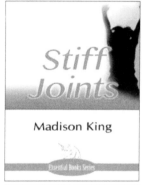

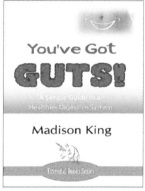
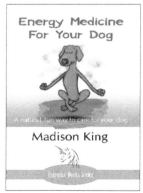